HOW TO GET YOURSELF TO STAY ON ANY DIET

Books by Charles F. Wetherall

Quit: Read This Book and Stop Smoking Forever
Diet: Read This Book and Stay Slim Forever
Winter Weightloss and Fitness Guide
Quit II: A Quit Smoking Guide for Women Only
How to Get Someone You Love to Stop Smoking
Kicking the Coffee Habit
The Gifted Kids Guide to Creative Thinking
The Gifted Kids Guide to Puzzles and Mind Games

CHARLES F. WETHERALL

HOW TO GET YOURSELF TO STAY ON ANY DIET

Andrews and McMeel
Universal Press Syndicate Company
Kansas City • New York

Library of Congress Cataloging-in-Publication Data

Wetherall, Charles F.
  How to get yourself to stay on any diet.

  1. Dieting.   2. Willpower.   3. Psychology.

ISBN: 0-8362-2414   87-91248

*If you could find a plan that could
build willpower and help you to win
the weight-loss battle once and for all—
would you read it?*

Of course, you would.

Well this is it!

How to Get Yourself to Stay on Any Diet
is just the plan you need.

*Read it and start your program to become
forever thin today!*

CONTENTS

INTRODUCTION

(Commonly referred to as that part of the book nobody reads)

This is a book about dieting. But if you've picked it up thinking it contains another miracle diet plan, you'll have to look elsewhere. I have no wonder diets nor magic menus on these pages.

Yes, there is some magic to be found here, but you'll discover that the magic is within yourself, just waiting to be discovered. You need only say the right word, the *abracadabra*, and your dieting dreams can come true.

But before you can make that happen, you'll need some answers. Some *real* answers. That's why I wrote this book. I wanted some answers to the dieting mystery. I wanted to know why, for example, when everybody is using mostly the same diets, some dieters win, whereas others fail. Why can one dieter pick up the *Pritikin Promise* or the *Rotation Diet*, lose weight and keep it off, but another dieter can try the *same* plans and reap nothing for his/her effort but failure and despair?

Why do forty-eight million dieters each year fail to stick to their diets and, therefore, lose the dieting battle? Why do one or two million win? Why not fifteen million and thirty-five million? Or forty and ten? What *really* separates the winners from the losers except for twenty or more pounds of ugly fat?

To be sure, I already had a glimmer of the answer prior to writing this book. I had successfully quit several unwanted habits and had written several best-selling books which showed others how to take charge of their lives and do the same. In the process of writing these works, I had the unenviable task of reading literally thousands of professional research studies. I've also read dozens of books on "quitting techniques" and behavior modification. But the answer I was looking for was not to be found on these lifeless pages of prose.

Instead, it was my interviews with successful dieters which pointed me in the right direction.

Over the years I have interviewed hundreds of people who have dieted and lost weight, who have quit smoking cigarettes or drinking coffee, who have stopped using alcohol or other dangerous drugs. Time and again these winners have proved to me that while "quitting technique" is an important ingredient in kicking any bad habit, it's a special power from *within* that produces ultimate success. To be more specific, it's not a better *diet* that sets the overweight free from the tyranny of unwanted fat. It's better *doit*.

In a word, the abracadabra, if you will, is *willpower*.

No, I'm not talking about that ordinary sort of willpower that well-meaning people, the professional and hoi polloi alike, think about when the word "willpower" is mentioned. You know, "moral fiber," "backbone," that sort of rubbish. I'm talking about that dynamic mental power that learned psychologists and philosophers have for centuries told us is the single, most important ingredient in achieving personal success; that one quality which, more than any other, separates winners from losers.

I know. I used to be one of the losers. For years I dieted. Most times I'd drop out after a couple of weeks. Sometimes I would quit after a couple of days. More than once I've quit my diet after a few *hours*. The word "permanent" was never part of my dieting vocabulary.

But I deeply wanted to be done with the misery of dieting *once and for all*. And that meant making permanent changes in my eating behavior, changes I had heretofore been unable to make. I simply lacked the willpower to do so.

Taking a lead from the successful dieters I had interviewed, I stopped reading research studies and started learning the principles of how to build willpower. I learned that successful men and women have been using willpower building exercises since the dawn of recorded history but never before have these methods been developed specifically for *dieters*. The more I read, the more convinced I was that these exercises could provide modern dieters with the tools they need to finally win the weight-loss battle. I updated these exercises and developed new ones. And the results have been remarkable.

Now I have a useful skill which enables me to control *all* aspects of my life. I can easily stick to any diet I want (in the unlikely event that I will ever diet again). I can persist in any undertaking I desire. I can succeed whenever I want, and on my own terms, not someone else's.

I'm teaching others how to do the same in my successful Weight Loss Through Willpower seminars. And this book can teach you these wonderful principles, too.

No, it doesn't offer another fad or crash diet to try your patience. It offers a proven program that could change your life forever. If you can read this sentence, you can change the dreadful odds you take into the weight-loss wars. No matter how many diets you've tried and failed, you can win, once and for all. Trust me. And become thin again.

Good luck.

C.F.W.

*The fault is not
in our stars,
but in ourselves,
that we are
underlings.*

—William Shakespeare

1

Permanent Weight Loss and the Elusive Silver Bullet

It usually begins something like this:

One morning after you shower, your eye is caught by the partially nude body staring back at you from a foggy bathroom mirror. However poorly the glass mirrors intimate detail, it still clearly reflects the broad outlines of your gluttonous sin. Once again you've created far more flesh than your frame can respectfully support.

Fat that's oozing from your bra or bulging from your shorts. Fat that grotesquely distends your thighs. Fat that sags from your stomach and droops from your chin, your fanny and arms.

Reluctantly, you step to a scale dusty from disuse to confront your suspicions. And there it is, reported in steely-cold facts more candid than even your most critical glance would have revealed: You're really overweight. *Again*. And it's only been two months since you were on your last diet. No, you didn't reach your goal but you did lose "some" weight. At least enough so you could tell yourself that you were thinner than you used to be.

But now you're decidedly crushed. You had pledged to yourself that *last* time was the last time. And now here you are again, facing the same dour parade of diet pills and a lifeless regimen of cottage cheese, dry toast, and low calorie "diet" meals.

Despite the grim forecast, you make the *Dieting Decision* so lightning fast that your lips are moving only milliseconds after your mind has privately intoned, "I've just got to go on a diet."

"What the heck," you now say aloud, "I've dieted before. I can do it again. Right?" But even as you renew your dieting pledge, you wonder whether you can really pull it off. Can you stick to your diet and stay thin? And you'll never know that, of course, until you try, try again.

Having made short work of the dieting decision, you are now ready for the next step in your fight to achieve the ideal figure: finding the diet plan that works. We all know what that is. That's the diet that's easy to stick to, yet reduces your weight; the plan that asks only minor concessions from your daily life; the plan that lets you eat cookies and chocolate malts but is *guaranteed* to keep fat off forever.

Although we all know that diet doesn't exist, we still keep looking. And from here the dieting scenario, reduced to its essential form, usually goes something like this:

Act I: The Search Begins

Your first stop is your home bookcase. The shelves fairly buckle under the weight of these previous weight-loss attempts. It's a virtual thesaurus of dieting despair. There was The Five-Day Wonder Diet, The Seven-Day Wonder Diet, The High Carb/Low Protein Diet, The High Protein/Low Carb Diet, The Metabolic Diet, and so on. Most of the books are so new-looking that a less scrupulous dieter could return them to the bookstore for full credit.

You've tried all these diets, if only briefly, and they've repaid you in the going currency of the dieting culture: You lost exactly the number of pounds that you so dearly paid for with their calorie-restricting menus.

But since you didn't *stay* on any of these diets, you didn't get what you ultimately wanted: a body so curvaceously thin it rivals the likes of such iconic images as Jane Fonda or Jim Palmer. So, the search goes on and you seek the counsel of friends. Friends are always eager to offer you advice. Their advice doesn't usually work, but at least it's free.

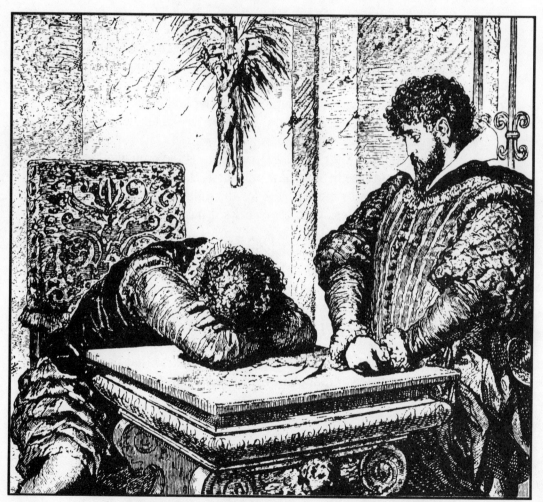

It's hell being told you have to go on another diet.

"Have you tried fasting?" Paula asks. "I heard you can lose weight really fast (no pun intended, she assures you). And the book says you don't even feel hungry after a couple of days."

You haven't tried fasting, but it sounds so extreme. I mean, would you trust something called *The Gandhi Diet?*

Then Paula recommends *Dr. Butler's 30-Day Can't-Miss Diet Plan* that she read about in the newspaper. But before she can explain it, Beth contradicts that the only way to get thin and stay thin is "Behavior Mod."

"You've got to *change* the way you eat," Beth says. "Otherwise, you'll never stay thin. You'll just gain it all back." Beth once weighed 165 pounds and dieted till she was a size 3. And you know, she was right. Although she started eating again she only gained *half* of it back (so far).

Charlie offers another solution. "Try the Metabolic Diet. I tried it and it's fantastic! I did it for three weeks and lost ten pounds."

Dick interjects that the Grapefruit Plan is the only way to go. "You buy these little yellow pills for $29.95. If they don't work, you get your money back for the pills you don't use. I got mine back in less than two weeks. I mean, how can you lose?"

As you consider the profundity of that notion, Barbara counters with another idea. "I saw a doctor on TV last week who had a whole new weight-loss idea that doesn't use diets at all. And it sounded so sensible, so easy. The doctor said that everybody has a certain weight at which they tend to stay. A 'setpoint' they call it. And no matter how much we diet, our body weight automatically keeps coming back to that point. The trick is to lower that point with *exercise*. Maybe that's the plan that can work for you."

You chat amiably about Barbara's Setpoint Plan but your mind fades back to the time you tried a Jane Fonda workout. You got aches and pains in places you didn't even know you had muscles. Besides, what with Billy's piano lessons and your new job, you just couldn't fit *regular* exercise into your schedule.

What Your Doctor Says

Confused, you turn to the experts. Obviously, if your family doctor doesn't have the answer, nobody does. The doctor says that it's not easy to lose weight (funny you didn't think of that), but says you can if you really try.

"Set realistic goals," he admonishes. "It's up to you," he says in parting, "I can't do it for you. That'll be $50. Next!"

You're admittedly dissatisfied with that advice. You've just blown fifty bucks to hear an M.D. parrot something you could have read for nothing in any magazine in the doctor's waiting room. What you really wanted was some *new* dieting intelligence. A silver bullet, as it were. Some new pill or potion, a "calorie blocker" that in one wave of the magic wand will leave you forever thin. Undaunted, you head to the clubrooms of all dieting America, the local bookstore.

The Dieting Cognoscenti

Wow! Have you ever seen so many diet books in all your life? It's absolutely boggling! There's a diet plan for every whim, every mood, every day of the year.

It seems that *everyone* has written a diet book. Doctors, movie stars, movie has-beens, nutritionists, clinicians, rock musicians, scientists, self-appointed experts, exercise physiologists, psychiatrists, dentists, the whole lot. Yes, even *Gandhi* has written a diet book. In fact, there are so many diet books that you'd need a year's worth of Sunday book review sections just to keep their titles straight.

Fortunately for you, Paula has already read the reviews and recommended *Dr. Butler's 30-Day Can't-Miss Diet Plan*. And now, face-to-face with its slick cover and glossy promises, you fork over $10.95 and get ready to try again.

Act II: Down the Up Staircase

Now comes the fun part. You begin Dr. B's 30-DCMDP *allegro vivace;* your willpower propelled by a reservoir hip-deep in memories of unwanted eating behavior; your bingeing, your gluttony, your unsightly figure. Your desire to become slim and stay that way is vigorous and strong. Your dieting concentration is keen and sharp. Your dedication to succeed is at a fever pitch.

As the days pass, the pounds go tripping by. First three pounds. Then another pound. And another. Soon you've lost nine pounds. Almost as if by magic, you march toward a slimmer, more youthful you. You can *feel* it in the way your clothes relax their relentless clutch. You can actually *see* it in the mirror you're now willing to face without shame or guilt. And this diet is *easy* to follow. In fact, you're sailing along so nicely it's almost too good to be true.

And you're right.

Act III: Up the Down Staircase

At this point in your dieting drama, subtle changes start seeping into your diet and your life. You have been dutifully sticking to those twelve-hundred-calorie menus when dieting starts to lose its appeal. The pounds aren't dropping as fast as they used to. Dr. B's menus are getting exponentially more boring with each passing plate of cottage cheese and bowl of butterless popcorn. Your desire to continue dieting begins to fade, and with it, your ability to pay attention to the daily dieting regime.

About this time, a quiet voice starts whispering those naughty little messages in your ear. Mysterious voices that tell you to start cheating: "Wouldn't a nice pan of brownies taste good right now?"

You return to your diet books for help. But they're virtually cover-to-cover recipes. You can also find the calorie content of everything from abalone to zwieback, but not a word on how to shore up a faltering willpower. And let's face it, by this time you need a hot fudge malt and a cheeseburger so badly your hair hurts.

As you bravely march onward, you find that these renegade cravings grow stronger, fed by the sugar and salt of daily life:

Your boss chews you out for being late. You're mad.

Your boss gives you a raise. You're glad.

The family cat dies. You're sad.

Your spouse cracks up the family car. You're grounded.

You gain three pounds when you should have lost one. You're disheartened.

You get tired of dieting. You're bored.

Your son gets caught smoking pot in the high school lavatory. You're livid.

The house payment is two months past due. You're scared.

It's the holiday season. You want to eat, drink, and be merry.

At the beginning of your diet, you successfully deflected these annoying intrusions without caloric malfeasance. But as time goes on (and God knows time is certainly on the side of dieting enemies, isn't it?), these nettlesome barbs start poking serious fissures in your willpower. Soon, those maverick little sentences grow into blazing statements of belligerent indifference. "I've been good, one little treat won't hurt." "I just don't think I want to diet anymore."

"Wouldn't a nice hot pan of brownies taste good right now?"

And now here you are having lunch with friends who have thoughtlessly told the waitress to bring a round of desserts for everyone. You are face-to-face with the enemy: a slab of hot apple pie embellished with a shovelful of creamy smooth cinnamon ice cream.

"Should I, or shouldn't I?" That is the question as you teeter on the brink of dieting mortality. "I mustn't let go," you plead to yourself. "Willpower, don't flake out on me now," you beg.

But you don't stand a chance against an enemy that has

been making a doily of your willpower with its relentless cunning and wile. "I'll get back on my diet tomorrow," you promise yourself, and then with lusty abandon you join your friends in perfidious delight.

The next day you're in the grocery store and you discover that beneath all those fresh fruits and colorful vegetables, you've quietly slipped a pint of your favorite premium ice cream. And a package of cookies. And perhaps another of your old friends. You try not to think about what you're doing. About the diet that's slipping away. It would only add to the guilt.

But the enemy knows your willpower is treading psychological water. And emboldened by yesterday's success it seizes the moment and sends your diet and your willpower into a maelstrom of guilt, confusion and unbridled appetite.

In the coming days you try to straighten yourself out and get back on the diet track. But you find your desire to diet is inversely related to every bite of forbidden food: the more you eat, the less you want to diet. It's so hard, you complain. Dieting seems like such a waste of time. And you never win. So you decide to wait. Regroup forces later on. Try again some other day.

And as the final curtain comes down you play your big scene. There you are, alone in the kitchen, acting with characteristic flourish. Eating with the kind of bingeful disregard that regains every pound you ever lost, plus a few more as added incentive for your next performance. Neither Meryl Streep nor Sir Laurence Olivier could have done it better.

Prologue

Well, there you have it. Another three-act dieting play with an ending as predictable as a Saturday night sitcom. The heroic start. The initial successes. Then "something" happens and your willpower vanishes just as surely as ice cream melts on Texas sidewalks.

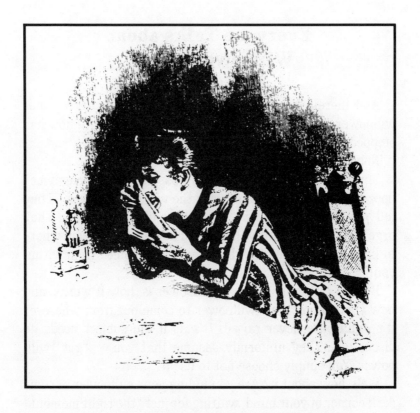

Is Your Next Diet Doomed?

You have doubtless participated in this dieting drama so many times that you can't count them all. And surely by now you must be asking yourself, "What's wrong with me? Why is my willpower so strong at the *beginning* of my diet but so wimpy later on? Where is my willpower when I need it most? Why can't I stay on a diet like I see other people do? Am I doing something wrong? And if I correct that 'something' can I win the trim, graceful figure I've always wanted?"

Millions of dieters, just like yourself, are as bewildered as you by their seeming lack of willpower and inability to stick to a diet; by the welter of conflicting weight-loss programs which promise so much and produce so little. They're looking for some answers. Some *real* answers.

Everyone Talks about
Willpower but . . .

And therein lies the problem: most everyone agrees that willpower is crucial to dieting success, but who until now has stepped forward to tell you how to get it?

Nobody.

Sure, dieting books and weight-loss articles in magazines liberally season their pages with the word "willpower." They tell you that willpower is "crucial" to dieting success. They urge you to "use" your willpower. They'll even tell you where to find it: The discipline, they say, has to come "from within you."

But the questions of what willpower *is*, how it works, and how you can get your willpower to come out from wherever it's hiding are never raised. It's as if the subject needs no discussion. They uniformly assume that you've "got" willpower. You simply choose not to use it.

Well, how about it? Are you hiding your willpower in some dark corner of your mind, waiting for just "the right moment" to unleash its dictatorial fury? I think not. Because the facts prove otherwise.

Half of the U.S. population—seventy-nine million adults—is overweight. Each year, some fifty million overweight men and women go on diets just like Ms. Everydieter in the scenario you've just read. But virtually every one of them, more than ninety-five percent, fail to muster the willpower they need to stick to their diets. If they had a strong, effective willpower, surely they would use it, wouldn't they? Wouldn't you?

Well, not necessarily. Dieters have willpower. They just don't know how to use it.

"It is will, force of purpose," said psychologist William Atkinson, "that enables us to do whatever we set our mind upon doing. He who resolves upon doing a thing," he added, "by that very resolution often scales the barriers to it, and secures its achievement."

English statesman and author Benjamin Disraeli agreed. "I have brought myself by long meditation to the conviction that a human being with a settled purpose must accomplish it, and that nothing can resist a will which will stake even existence upon its fulfillment."

Or as contemporary willpower scientist Dr. Robert Assagioli has said, "The training and use of willpower is the foundation of all endeavors."

Apples and Oranges

While these quotes may sound like typical historical overstatement which could be spoken in the same persuasive breath as "I have but one life to give to my country," they're really not overstating their case at all. That's because Assagioli and his learned colleagues are not talking about the sort of dime store willpower to which most dieting books and magazines pay glancing lip service. They're not talking about "moral fiber" or that iron-willed determination nonsense that comes to most minds when the word "willpower" is mentioned.

They're talking about real, honest-to-goodness willpower: a complex, multifaceted mental power than can be organized, exercised, and strengthened to help men and women achieve *any* goal they desire. And the difference between this kind of willpower and that cardboard caricature of the popular press is the difference between success and failure, rich and poor, win or lose, and above all, fat or thin.

Willpower Can Make Your Dreams Come True

A trained willpower is one of the mind's most wondrous faculties. It can blend the appetites and passions of the physical body with the miraculous power and forces of the mind into one harmonious whole.

A fully developed willpower allows you to determine just what suggestions control your thoughts, emotions, and actions, instead of leaving yourself prey to reckless impulse or chance circumstance.

A well-trained willpower operates freely and instinctively in all phases of your life. It can solve the petty annoyances of your life, as well as the major challenges. It can help you achieve your goals, no matter what you conceive them to be: a more assertive manner, quitting smoking, earning a million dollars, or losing weight permanently.

Willpower can do all this and more. If you understand what willpower is, how it works, and most importantly, how you

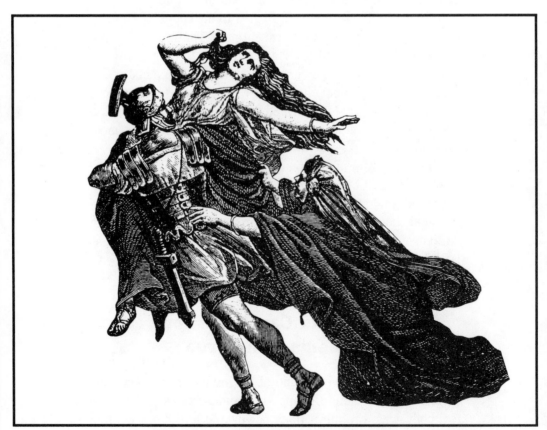

Being thin has its obvious disadvantages.

can *build* willpower, I can guarantee that your weight-loss problems will be over.

Your Journey to a Perfect Size

This book is going to help you do just that. I'll teach you how to harness this awesome power and put it to work in your dieting life. Once organized and strengthened, willpower can set you free from the maddening, fruitless search for the diet that works. And there's really nothing mysterious about it at all.

Here's what I'm going to do. Building willpower is as simple as one, two, three. If you follow these proven steps, you'll develop—often in thirty days or less—the willpower you need to win with *any* diet you choose.

First, I'll teach you what willpower is and how it works.

Then, I'll show you how to evaluate your willpower. I'll teach you what parts of your willpower are strong, which are weak and letting you down.

Finally, I'll teach you how to *build* willpower through more than twenty proven exercises. With a strong, well-trained will, you can stick to your diet and stay slim for as long as you like.

Does all this sound too good to be true? Well, there is a catch. You're going to have to work at it. In dieting as in life, there are no free rides. I'm not peddling magic formulas in which you give ten cents' worth of effort and get back two bucks in weight loss. This plan is strictly *quid pro quo*, something for something.

On the other hand, these exercises call for no hard labor and no huge sacrifice. You need no great amount of education. All it takes is a certain willingness to succeed, and since this is a book about building willpower, you'll have plenty of opportunities to build this willingness even if you don't possess it now.

And one other thing. Don't mistake my sometimes lighthearted tone for any suggestion that I'm not serious about the subject. I know what it means to be fat. I know what it's like to blow diet after diet, to fail time after time.

But serious usually means boring. And since we've got too much boring in our lives already, why not lighten up as we lighten up? It is my hope this book will make both possible.

But wait no more. I lift my lamp beside the golden door.

*Never eat more
than you can lift.*

—Miss Piggy

The Willpower You Never Knew

I can think of no other word in the lexicon of dieting that has been so abused, so misunderstood, as willpower. Ask a person what "cat" means and you'll get a reasonably accurate description of that fuzzy little feline. But ask somebody what "willpower" is and you'll probably wind up with as many definitions as uses one waggish author has found for dead cats.

"Willpower is being able to see the reward of being thinner more clearly," wrote one of my willpower class students. Another said, "staying away from fattening foods and eating low-calorie food that is healthy." "Willpower is the will to succeed," said still another. "It's sticking to the diet or if I go off the diet, getting right back on it," says a fourth.

Actually, those definitions are fairly accurate since most people correctly believe that willpower helps control behavior. But it's a totally different story when you ask *how* willpower does whatever it does. Here, dieters and non-dieters alike enter the great black *terra incognitae.* And without knowledge of *how* willpower does what it does, you can imagine what kind of success dieters have in making willpower fulfill its mysterious mission.

The Gatekeeper Theory

Many people, for example, subscribe to what I call the *Great Gatekeeper* theory of willpower. According to this view of behavior control, willpower is a mental gatekeeper, a lonely sentinel someplace in the attic of your skull whose sole purpose is to prevent you from behaving unwisely.

When kicking unwanted habits, for example, "Igor" the Gatekeeper is supposed to stop you from smoking, or drinking, or chewing tobacco, or biting your nails, or resisting the sensual touch of a forbidden lover. Or whatever.

Dieters who view willpower in this way try to summon their willpower to help them resist the myriad temptations which inevitably accompany calorie-restricting diets.

"I've just *got* to get myself to stop eating," these dieters plead with themselves. "I just can't let myself go out of control." Sounds like war, doesn't it? And it is. Dieting is a mental war for these corpulent souls as their willpower ceaselessly collides with the forces of caloric wrongdoing.

The problem is that sheer willpower may *occasionally* be sufficient to stem the tide of ruthless temptation. But as you know, most of the time it either can't, or won't, give you the help you need and want. And that's because you're asking your willpower to do something which, in fact, it wasn't *designed* to do.

Willpower is not a mental power which you apply *directly* to control *unwanted* behavior. It is not steely-cold nerves, backbone, moral fiber, iron-willed determination, or any of those other willpower buzzwords. And it cannot be used to coerce yourself into being a good little boy or girl.

Will the Real Willpower Please Stand Up?

Instead, willpower is a dynamic, multifaceted energy that creates the conditions under which you can stick to your diet long enough to develop the new behavior to help you become permanently thin. And, with a little effort on your part, it's amenable to change, growth and remarkable improvement. Put in a handy working definition, it would look like this:

> *Willpower is a learned mental ability to control one's behavior through the direction of itself and other psychological forces.*

As you'll note, there are three major differences between this definition and the popular Gatekeeper notions about willpower.

Willpower Is a Learned Skill

The first is that willpower is a *learned* skill. You are not genetically programmed with some inalterable quantum of willpower to control your life. What you are given is the basic mental material, the building blocks, as it were, with which to *develop* willpower. In much the same way as we're given the mental equipment to think, to remember, to see, to feel, to taste, we learn to culture willpower and these other faculties through experience and training to be more responsive to our needs.

Yes, I'd agree that there may be slight differences in our innate willpower ability, just as there are modest differences in our ability to remember, to think clearly, to learn and discern. But these differences, whatever they may be, are not nearly so important as the enormous chasms that separate organized and unorganized willpowers.

Willpower Is a Director

Second, you'll notice that the responsibility of willpower has been mercifully shifted. Willpower is no longer described as the actual *doer* of self-control. Willpower is not bully power. It is not responsible for preventing you from, or making you do, anything. So you can stop beating yourself up because your willpower couldn't coerce you into behaving.

Willpower Has Help

Finally, you'll observe that willpower doesn't act alone. It is not a lonely sentinel. Willpower has help. But rather than directly controlling unwanted eating behavior, willpower regulates and directs *other* psychological forces which, in turn, control dieting behavior.

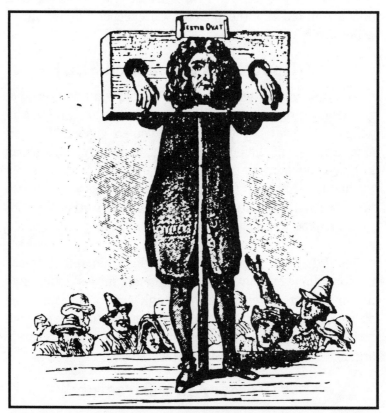

It was easy to stick to a diet in earlier days. Just insult the Crown and you're guaranteed to lose twenty pounds.

What kind of forces? Well, you're familiar with them all. The only difference is you've probably never thought of these powers as essential components of willpower. Forces like imagination, desire, emotions, concentration, persistence, and others. These are the forces which your willpower controls to *willfully* produce your every success, dieting or otherwise.

Getting a Fresh Start

To begin your dieting renaissance, I want you to forget your notions of willpower as some sort of one-dimensional mental chastity belt. Instead, think of willpower as simply *willing powerfully.* That is, willpower (1) chooses a course of action and then, (2) carries out that action powerfully. But when I say "powerfully," I mean a willpower which exhibits not one but *seven* readily identifiable attributes. Attributes that can be exercised and strengthened to stick to your diet.

SEVEN QUALITIES THAT MAKE WILLPOWER EFFECTIVE

1. Decisiveness

Any time you begin a diet, or use your willpower to make other salutary changes, you'll be confronted by conflicting goals which press for the status quo. Remember when you learned how to ride your bike? Sure you do. You fell down a lot, didn't you? We all did. But nicking shins or bloodying elbows are part of the conflicting goals in your adolescent life that you resolved. That is, you agreed that the long-term goal of learning how to ride a bicycle was more important than the short-term goal of a childhood *without* skinned knees, torn trousers and a bruised ego.

Moving up the ladder of life, we learned that the goal of

dating and marriage was probably a far better goal than the competing goal of the peace and serenity which come from a dateless life where one is never rejected, cheated upon, or given some cruddy venereal disease.

Dieting also produces conflicting goals. Yes, it's nice to become thin but conflicting goals fight for the status quo. Certainly when you cut your calorie intake to twelve hundred or less per day you'll raise havoc with your goal of physiological and psychological peace and tranquility. Let's face it. It's fun to eat anything you want and nobody can say it isn't.

You'll also confront your desire to look and feel less like a spoilsport when you're lunching with friends, as well as your need for a normal, more hassle-free life which is almost dichotomous with dieting.

And what about exercise? Sheer inertia implores us to delay it or forget it altogether. Rainy days and busy schedules can make sitting home and relaxing an attractive alternative.

Since it's quite literally impossible to have your cake and eat it too, willpower decisiveness reconciles these various competitive urges into a unified agreement. That is, you *decide* whether or not to actually attempt to attain the goal, given the known barriers to its achievement.

While this decision-making process sounds simple, it's easily the single most important stage of willing. Dieters often cannot stick to their diets because they failed to accept the crucial difference between *complying* with a diet and *surrendering* to one; the difference between half-hearted dieting attempts and supreme efforts with unflagging persistence.

The difference may have seemed trifling to you but decisiveness is easily the most important willpower step of all. You'll soon learn that almost supernatural dieting willpower can be yours when you truly surrender to the dieting formula.

2. Strength

Strength of willpower is certainly the best known of all willpower attributes, although it's by no means the most important. Strength of will is that quality which the layman almost always ascribes to will. In fact, most people mistakenly believe that strength *is* willpower. And it's belief in this truncated version of willpower that produces much of the failure when dieters go jowl-to-jowl with temptation.

Dieters with strong willpower can restrain an impulse directed toward an immediate pleasure in favor of some greater satisfaction that is removed by distance in time or space. In table language, that means skipping the pie à la mode so you can earn a slim, graceful body in the weeks ahead.

The ability to say "No!" to tempting, high-calorie treats is obviously important to the dieter. But this skill is really not

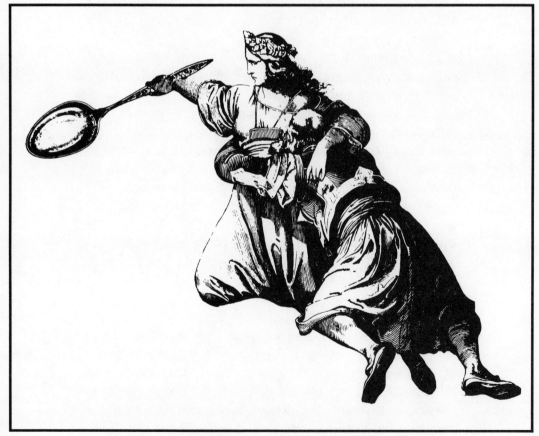

"But I simply MUST have a dish of chocolate ice cream!"

your first line of willpower defense. Important as strength of willpower is, it's virtually useless without other, more important qualities of will. Unless guided, restrained, tempered, and intensified by the other qualities, strength of willpower is—naked and alone—about as effective as a spaceship without a guidance system, an automobile without a steering wheel, Tammy Bakker without mascara.

3. Intensity

Intensity is the degree of *energy* which your willpower uses to accomplish its desired ends. You might say it's your willpower voltage. It's the direct result of desire, an emotional eagerness or excitement of the mind directed toward the attainment of your goal. As such, desire is precedent to every action of willpower.

This dynamic force, when fanned by the psychological flames of imagination, creates the energy your willpower needs to achieve any task you set before it.

If you are to be successful at losing weight, your reasons for dieting and exercising must be forceful and compelling; your commitment must be deep and genuine. You must want to lose weight permanently. You must want this goal earnestly, actively, vigorously, constantly, and persistently.

Unfortunately, the desire to achieve weight-loss goals can easily be dimmed by many factors, including your ability to concentrate on dieting success. And that's why you need to develop skills to maintain your desire and provide your willpower with the fuel it needs.

4. Concentration

Concentration is the ability to keep your attention focused on your dieting goal and the related psychological forces which make reaching that goal possible. What I'm talking about here is not only the ability to remember from one day to the next that you're on a diet and to concentrate your attention on meal planning, calorie counting and the rest of the dieting regimen. I'm also talking about your ability to hold

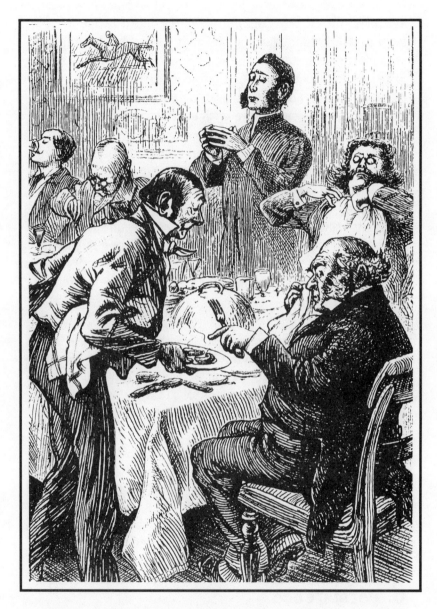

before your mind the psychological forces I've just mentioned to improve your dieting success.

Italian psychologist Roberto Assagioli compares the function of concentration to that of the lens which focuses rays of the sun, concentrating and intensifying the heat. Just as the lens magnifies the strength of the sun, concentration magnifies the strength of your willpower. It does so by its ability to produce and maintain in the mind the various psychological forces at its disposal: imagination, desire, emotions, etc. The result of this concentration is that wills of only moderate strength can succeed where without this concentration they may have failed.

Many dieters find that their willpower is effective in producing concentration only at the beginning of a diet. This is often because their desire to succeed is strong. But when non-dieting problems invade their lives, the goal of losing weight is crowded from immediate view and eventually lost in the psychological shuffle. Their focus of attention is blurred. The magnifying power of their lens of concentration is muddied. And a significant, if not fatal, reduction of their strength of willpower results.

5. Confidence

Sure you want to become thin. But do you have the self-confidence to achieve it? For most dieters, this is no small consideration. They have tried dozens of diet plans but failed every time to stick to their program, reach their goal, and stay slim forever.

The result of repeated failure is that many dieters begin to unconsciously think of themselves not as dieters who have failed, but as dieting *failures*. They might even openly question their ability to lose weight permanently, so serious are their doubts about their ability to succeed. Embracing this emotional mindset, their doubts become a self-fulfilling prophecy.

6. Persistence

This is one of my favorite qualities of willpower. It is, I think, the most crucial of all willpower components since in the final analysis, the ability to *stick to* your diet turns continuing weight losses—regardless of how small—into eventual victory.

Dieters typically start a diet, stay on it for a few weeks or so, but when one of the willpower attributes fades, they quit. Then, after a few months of creeping weight gains and growing guilt, they pick up the torch and try again, usually driven more by hope for success than convincing new plans or techniques to achieve it.

Persistence is the willpower attribute that gets these dieters back on the dieting wagon. Despite temporary setbacks, despite demoralizing failures, persistent dieters hold to their calling until victory has been achieved.

7. Control

Control is the ability to "operate" the various qualities of willpower and the psychological forces upon which willpower often depends. When your willpower is trained and organized, it can control itself and invoke the other psychological forces at the right time, in the right proportions, and in the proper way to produce a favorable result.

When a particular quality of willpower—strength, for example—does not produce the desired result (and many times it does not), the well-trained willpower can easily choose a *combination* of forces to achieve its purpose. Maybe strength, concentration, and increased desire are a more workable grouping. Or perhaps a team of persistence and desire. In fact, the whole notion of effective willpower is the art of harnessing a selected *team* of attributes to produce a successful result.

That's what you're learning how to do in this book. It's your owner's guide to the care, feeding and operation of your willpower.

Putting It All Together

Well, there you have it. That wasn't so mysterious, was it? Seven simple yardsticks which we use to measure the well-trained willpower. Now let's see what they look like in action, with this brief nondieting display.

I have a fourteen-year-old son who is a walking billboard for willpower in action. Marty is like many kids his age, kids who become obsessed with some sport or activity. When he was a grade-schooler, it was dinosaurs. Then it was rock music. Now Marty's obsession of choice is tennis. And in this one area, his willpower attributes stand out in remarkable contrast for easy viewing and comparison.

To say that Marty likes tennis is to say that the pope's hobby is Catholicism or that it occasionally gets cold in Minnesota. Marty *loves* tennis. He eats, sleeps, and breathes tennis. And his willpower works wonders to help him achieve his goal: to become the best tennis player he can be. All this despite the fact that he's largely oblivious to operations of his willpower. That's an important point and I'll come back to it.

Marty plays tennis virtually every day. About the only days in season when he doesn't play are when it rains or snows (in Minnesota we usually have to shovel snow from the outdoor courts starting in September. We don't have to shovel the indoor courts until February) or when he's sick (and I mean *really* sick).

Marty takes tennis lessons. He found his own instructor, and he also found himself an on-going tennis program so he can compete with other players his age and skill level. He frequently plays in neighborhood tournaments, testing and improving his skills, monitoring his abilities, building his confidence.

Marty is a member of his high school tennis team. Many of his friends are kids he plays tennis with, both team and non-team members.

Marty frequently visits tennis and other athletic stores to look, feel, smell, and virtually drink up every last ounce of tennis intelligence (I call it trivia) he can find. He's always got his eye on the next tennis racket he'll buy (with his own money, too).

Since Marty doesn't drive yet, I'm his chauffeur. And on these weekly jock stops, I usually wind up in the corner looking at clothes while he gets into learned discussions with the shop pros about some arcane tennis nuance: the handling characteristics of ceramic rackets versus graphite; increasing top-spin by changing string tension. That sort of thing. Most of the time I don't even know what they're talking about.

This kid will watch TV tennis matches over virtually anything else on the tube. And often when the commercials run, he's mentally and physically trying out new shots against imaginary living room opponents. We've lost a few good lamps that way. And it's no accident that whenever I serve him up one of my kitten-soft, left-handed backhands on the real courts, he turns that fuzzy yellow ball into an unplayable ballistic missile with his cross-court backhand slice, a neat little tactic he picked up from his current TV idol, Boris Becker.

Marty reads about tennis. Books. Magazines. Newspaper articles. Tennis ball cans. Anything he can lay his hands on. And from his readings he develops his own strategies, mentally, on paper, and on the courts.

Where There's a Will . . .

In short, Marty is using his willpower the way all winners do, and by that I mean *all* of us. His voluminous reading builds his tennis skills by teaching him new tennis shots and strategies. But more importantly, it builds his desire and confidence. When he reads and vicariously participates in his books and magazines, he builds his desire to emulate the action of the printed page in his tennis life. He also learns about new tennis shots and strategies he wants (desires) to try.

He builds his *persistence* through his team membership, his choice of tennis-playing friends and record-keeping. His *concentration* is developed by his endless tennis participation, his internal and external goal setting, by use of his imagination and emotions. His *confidence* is bolstered by his successes, both in regular and tournament play. But even his failures steel his *desire* to "do better" next time. And his *strength* of willpower is augmented by his reading, his total immersion in his sport.

Do you see what I mean? His rabid interest in tennis is a *self-perpetuating* phenomenon. The more he plays tennis, watches tennis, reads about tennis, thinks about tennis, imagines about tennis, etc., the more he wants to play tennis, and the greater his ability to play tennis and reach his goal.

Now certainly you could argue with this interpretation by saying, "Sure he has willpower to become a good tennis player. He *likes* to play tennis. But dieting isn't like that. I don't *like* to diet and that's why it's so difficult to do. Try asking that kid of yours to clean up his room and see what kind of willpower he's got."

And I'd say that is precisely the point. And if you're reading this book with one of those big yellow or green highlight pens in your hand, get ready to paint a big swath through the next few sentences.

When we attempt to accomplish goals which have our *undivided* desire and unequivocable support, we use our willpower fully and appropriately to make that goal a reality.

But when we attempt to achieve goals which have less than our total support, like dieting, we become petulant foot-draggers. If we use our willpower at all, it's likely to be that sliver called strength of willpower. And using strength alone is like sending Mr. Peepers to Hulk Hogan's house for an afternoon of arm wrestling.

How Winners Use Willpower

Not so with the dieting winners. They use the full measure of their willpower without conscious strain or effort. In fact, one sure way to tell that a dieter is a winner is when he or she diets almost *effortlessly*. Notice I say "almost." After all, nothing worthwhile is easy.

Dieting winners read books and magazines on dieting and nutrition. Lots of them. Because they *want* to. They want to soak up as much knowledge as possible about their subject and how to achieve their goal.

Many of the winners belong (and attend) dieting clubs for

precisely the same reason as Marty belongs to his tennis club: They want to test and improve their dieting skills, monitor their abilities and progress, build their confidence, and find the support they need to persist in their dieting program.

Successful dieters hang around with successful dieters for the same reasons. Not because somebody told them it would be a nice idea ("Marty, I think it would be nice if you clean up your room before the cleaning lady comes"), but because they just *naturally* seek out the kind of people who share their interest and support.

The winners make vivid use of their psychological power of imagination to build their willpower desire. They hang photos of their former skinny selves on refrigerator doors; they window shop for the clothes they'll soon be wearing because they stick to their diet; they *imagine* what it's going to be like to be thin, alive, *active*.

Dieters who use their willpower properly often seek their own dieting answers and develop their own dieting strategies. They don't turn their will and their lives over to the likes of the Pritikens, the Simmons, or the Katahns of the world. They find their own answers to the dieting dilemma.

And that's just the beginning.

Look to Yourself to Find a Winner

Still have that Magic Marker? Then underline this:

> *Every single person reading this book has willpower.*

Everyone of you has successfully used your willpower in the past. Otherwise you couldn't have overcome the endless variety of challenges which have confronted you in the past:

finishing school or college, first loves, finding a lifetime mate, making tough career choices, finding new jobs, and so on. We have come a long way with our willpower. We are not habitual quitters and it's good to remember that.

But when it comes to sticking to a diet, dieters choke up. Because we don't *want* to diet, we do as little as possible. We neglect those wonderful willpower qualities we possess and which we have successfully used so many times before. Instead, we drag out this cardboard imitation and ask it to behave like some comic book superhero.

And if you're ever in doubt as to whether you're playing games with yourself on this issue, just ask yourself Wetherall's Question: "If a person *really wanted* to stick to a diet, what would that person do?"

Students in my weight-loss classes love this question. It allows them to freely brainstorm for answers without the necessity of committing themselves. I'm sure you know what happens. Because they're designing a program for somebody else, for somebody who "really wants" to stick to a diet, they instantly develop creative plans and innovative procedures which embrace all components of willpower: desire, imagination, emotions, concentration, confidence, persistence, the whole nine yards. That's why I say, willpower, left to its own devices, will succeed every time. It's when we attempt to *force* ourselves to do something that we come up losers.

That's why dieters don't win.

And that's what this book teaches. It shows you how to get yourself to use the full measure of your willpower. It shows you how to do on purpose what you have so many times successfully done before, without ever thinking about it. Except I'll show you how to do it *better*.

The Experts Think You Can

"It's quite clear that people can become thinner," says Dr. George Bray, of the Los Angeles County–University of South-

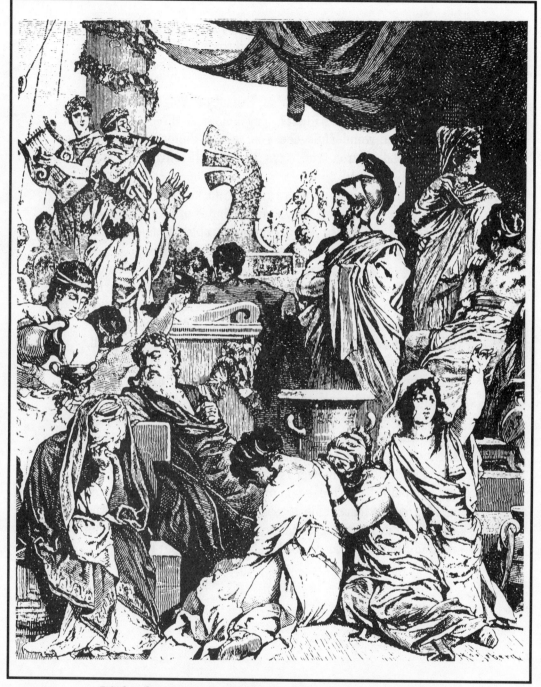

It's hard to stay on a diet when you're having a good time.

ern California Medical Center, "if they want to. And there's the rub. It may not be a failure of will that puts weight on, but an enormous amount of willpower is needed to take, and keep, pounds off."

Dieting expert Dr. Richard B. Stuart of Weight Watchers International agrees. Stuart, psychological director of the weight-loss group, says the goal of all dieters should be effective self-control. And, says Stuart, self-control is a skill that can be *learned*.

That's precisely what we're going to do, starting right now. First, we've got to find out which attributes of your willpower are strong, and which are giving you problems. And we can do that with the simple test on the following pages.

Then you'll begin a program to build effective willpower which includes more than fifteen proven exercises. I've tried to arrange these exercises in such a way as to put into motion only that part of your willpower "muscle" which is weak.

A number of exercises, for example, build strength of will, and ultimately, your ability to execute your diet. Others build decisiveness, confidence, persistence, concentration, and intensity. I would recommend that you first read this book entirely. Then, go back and carefully reread each chapter doing the exercises it prescribes and chart your progress on the log pages at the end of the book. You will find that in no time at all, your willpower is shouldering heavier loads without complaint. Sacrifices you previously thought were impossible are now not only possible, but actually *easy*. And complete dieting success, where it was formerly just a chimerical mirage, will begin to take shape as a visual reality.

*Every diet carries with it
the seeds of
failure or success.
Whether you win or lose
is largely a matter of
your own will.
And where there's a will,
there's a way.*

Where Is Your Willpower Letting You Down?

Getting a handle on the willpower attributes might seem a trifle complicated at first, especially in the dialectic of the printed page. But what it all boils down to is this:

Most dieters errantly believe that strength of willpower *is* willpower, and that this strength can be directly imposed on behavior. But when the acid test of caloric temptation confronts the unorganized will, they sit there like a bump on a log and try to tough it out using pure strength of willpower alone. Trouble is, you know as well as I do that no amount of iron-willed determination seems to withstand the enemy onslaught. Dieters instead should invoke all *seven* attributes of willpower *indirectly* to influence behavior.

The Operation of Will

Dr. Roberto Assagioli in his book *The Act of Will* makes an important contribution to understanding these two crucial points with this useful analogy:

The dieter who believes strength of willpower *is* willpower, says Assagioli, is like the motorist who gets into her car, starts the engine, releases the hand brake, and then gets out and tries to *push* her car. That's using willpower, all right, but in such a way that fails to accomplish its intended purpose. And yet this is precisely what dieters who cannot stick to their diets are doing. They attempt to force themselves to stay on their diet through sheer strength and determination. And it just doesn't work.

How much better it would be if the motorist got into her car, put the machine in gear, and thereafter *directed* and *regulated* the full range of her equipment to move the car to its destination.

What dieters ought to do is put their willpower in gear. Willpower mediates the transference of power beginning from selection of goal, through desire and the various supporting psychological functions into the finished product, a victorious diet. In other words, the smart dieter ought to do exactly what the smart motorist does.

1. She first chooses where she wants to go (or analogously, how much weight she wants to lose and for how long). This is her *goal*.

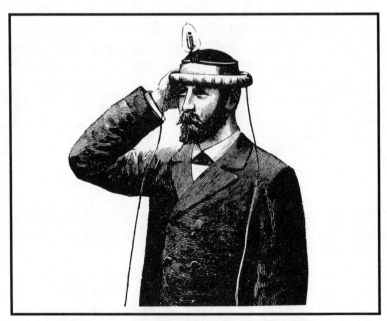

Man's first attempt at improving dieting willpower.

2. She reflects on her reasons for wanting to make the trip and balances that against her other goals which may conflict with her chosen ambition. She'll have to kennel her dog, for example, and she may not want to do that. She'll miss family and friends. They might be more important than her trip.

3. After deliberating on these various goals, she'll *decide* on the one most appropriate. And having exercised her decisiveness, she'll put the other goals out of sight for the time being.

4. She'll check to see whether she has sufficient *desire* to make her trip. And if she doesn't, her willpower will do something about it: she'll use her various psychological forces at her disposal to *build* willpower desire. She also keeps close accounting on her desire during her trip. And she frequently replenishes her supply as she goes forward to the finish line.

5. She *plans* her route. That is, just what dieting course she will take and how long it will take her to get there.

6. She *executes* her plan. No, she doesn't get out and push her car from New York to California. Nor does she try to force herself to behave. She puts her entire willpower into action. First, she gets her willpower in order. That's the psychological equivalent to getting a grease job, an oil change, checking the tires and battery, filling the car with gas, etc. That's what you're doing right now by reading this book.

Then, she gets into her dietary vehicle and starts the engine. She knows that if she's to successfully reach her destination she's got to operate her vehicle with the right controls. Just as she uses the brakes, gas pedal, steering wheel, headlights, etc., to guide her car, she uses her willpower controls—decisiveness, strength, desire, concentration, confidence, and persistence—to direct her dietary course. Moreover, she doesn't press on the gas when she wants to brake; she doesn't call for willpower "strength" when she really needs "persistence" or more "desire."

During her trip, she'll have to maneuver her diet around many obstacles, just as the motorist will, to stay on course. She will be confronted by a variety of warning signs and signals which demand her attention for a safe trip. She'll keep an eye on the gas gauge, for example, since it's a disheartening experience to run out of desire, the psychological fuel which makes your willpower run.

The Short Road Back

Few drivers who are determined to reach California will head back to the starting line when they run into a temporary roadblock in Indiana. Yet this is precisely what many dieters do. They run into a few obstacles and instead of trying to find alternative routes, they turn around and start the gluttonous trip back to Fat City whence they came.

Sure, there are setbacks. But what trip doesn't include a few wrong turns, maybe even a flat tire? Sometimes there are detours and dieting slips along her road. She may have to plow ruthlessly ahead to obviate some. On others she'll have to go the long way around instead of the most direct, though perhaps more dangerous, route.

And she'll avoid troublesome situations and locations. Since she has traveled this road many times, she knows in advance what and where these dangers lurk. And she doesn't take unnecessary chances.

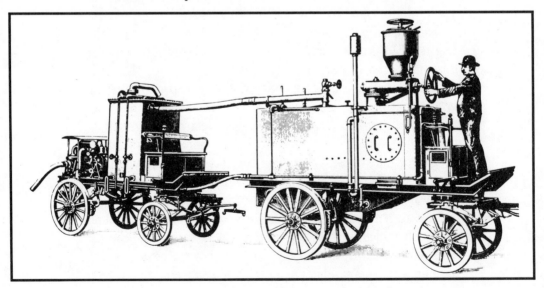

The Beginning Driver

On the other hand, if she's just learning to diet, the first few miles of the trip will be "stop and go" as she gets used to her plan and program. She'll be as unfamiliar with her new diet as she is with a strange country road or freeway in another city. Little by little, though, as she gains familiarity and expertise, the dieting program becomes second nature.

As dieting becomes natural, the subconscious takes over control. It knows the danger signals. It knows where she's going. It knows the important willpower tools she must use to keep her vehicle headed in the right direction.

If she does reach a temporary dead end, she doesn't sit there like a hapless twit. But she doesn't get out and try to push her dietary vehicle, either. Instead, through her training and experience, her willpower calls on the right forces in the right proportion to pull her out of this vulnerable spot.

Learning the Rules of the Road

All of this is spoken, however, as if you know precisely which attributes of your willpower are letting you down. And perhaps you do not.

I have interviewed thousands of people who have stayed on their diets, quit smoking, quit drinking coffee or alcohol, or stopped using other addictive chemicals. Uniformly, the reasons why they won their freedom were clothed in the form and fabric of willpower.

While few winners and losers knew the principles of willpower by name, they all spoke of their successes and failures as if "willpower" was their second language.

The losers reported their failures in terms of "lack of persistence" or "a loss of concentration," a failure to set "realistic" goals or, simply, an inability to say "no" to high-calorie treats.

Dieting winners spoke of their successes with phrases like,

"I finally made up my mind" (decisiveness), "I refused to think about food" (concentration), or "I was so determined to stay on this diet I wouldn't take 'no' for an answer" (desire).

Identifying Your Willpower Problems

Willpower attributes, unfortunately, don't come in airtight little boxes. They overlap themselves in effect and it's sometimes difficult to tell where the result of one leaves off and another begins.

For example, all dieters, of necessity, have more than one power of will which has failed and caused their dieting demise. Obviously, all dieters who fail to stick to their diets lack persistence, since persistence is just another way of saying you didn't stay on your diet. But dieters usually cite some other reason as the cause of their inability to be persistent; a personal problem, for example, or a bout with depression, nervousness, or anger.

You may also find that you had one or two reasons for goofing up one diet but find a different set as the reason you weren't able to stay on the next diet. For example, you may have found that sticking to a bizarre fad diet was physiologically too demanding, that you just couldn't keep your mind off "real" food long enough to win with that plan. Success on your next diet might have been sabotaged by personal problems or a lack of suitable progress.

Likewise, building decisiveness of willpower will likely increase the performance of *all* attributes of willpower. Similarly, a high degree of willpower *desire*, for example, may make up for a certain lack of concentration.

Nevertheless, it is helpful to know in which areas you are strong, and in which areas your willpower needs help so that you can devote the kind of specialized effort strong and effective willpower needs.

So grab a pencil and take a couple of minutes to carefully reflect on what shot down your previous diets. Be as honest and as thorough as you can. Fire when ready.

THE WILLPOWER TEST

Dieters fail to stick to their diets for a variety of reasons, most of them relating to the effectiveness of their willpower. Take a few moments and reflect upon your dieting history. Then, answer the following questions to determine which of these situations reflects your dieting experience.

1. Sometimes I have quit a diet without really knowing why. I just started eating again.

Yes ☐ No ☐

2. Oftentimes in past diets, I have been confronted with a favorite food and have been unable to resist it.

Yes ☐ No ☐

3. I have quit some dieting or exercise programs because they were too much work.

Yes ☐ No ☐

4. I often get to worrying so much about other things that I forget about my diet.

Yes ☐ No ☐

5. I have quit one or more diets because it seemed almost impossible to succeed.

Yes ☐ No ☐

6. I have quit diets because the discomfort associated with them was too much to bear.

Yes ☐ No ☐

7. When I diet, I often start arguing with myself and finally talk myself into cheating.

Yes ☐ No ☐

8. Losing weight permanently is important to me, but not so important that I would make changes in my life style.

Yes ☐ No ☐

9. I have sometimes gotten depressed over something and given up my diet. Somehow, the diet didn't seem important anymore.

Yes ☐ No ☐

10. Several times I have gotten close to my weight-loss goal, but gave up. Losing the last few pounds didn't seem important.

Yes ☐ No ☐

11. I often find myself thinking about food, and before long, I go off my diet.

Yes ☐ No ☐

12. There are times during past diets when I simply couldn't say "no" to a treat.

Yes ☐ No ☐

13. I change my mind frequently about starting and stopping my diet.

Yes ☐ No ☐

14. Sometimes I have given up on dieting because it just seemed as if I wasn't getting any thinner.

Yes ☐ No ☐

15. I am a typical "yo-yo" dieter. I lose some weight, then gain it back, then go on another diet.

Yes ☐ No ☐

16. I have a physical problem that makes it very difficult for me to lose weight.

Yes ☐ No ☐

17. When dieting, I often daydream about food and eating.

Yes ☐ No ☐

18. Reaching my ideal weight is important and I will do anything reasonable to achieve it.

Yes ☐ No ☐

19. I have so much weight to lose that I sometimes think it's impossible to lose it all.

Yes ☐ No ☐

20. If I cheat on my diet, I am likely to quit it altogether.

Yes ☐ No ☐

What Components of Your Willpower Need Help?

I've given this little quiz many times to students in my Weight Loss Through Willpower seminars. It isolates and identifies exactly which component of your willpower is giving you the most trouble.

ANSWERS

If You Answered "Yes" to These Questions	You Need Help with This Component of Willpower
1, 8, 13, 15	Decisiveness
2, 7, 12	Strength
3, 10, 18	Intensity (Desire)
4, 11, 17	Concentration
5, 9, 14, 19	Confidence
6, 16, 20	Persistence

Where to From Here?

As you look back over your answers keep the above key in mind. You'll readily see that the various weaknesses in willpower attributes cause various dieting problems to occur.

Most dieters who have taken this test have shown the most trouble with three willpower attributes: decisiveness, strength, and confidence. That hardly should be surprising. As I've said, most dieters failed because they haven't truly surrendered to the requirements of getting and staying thin: diet and exercise. And when they haven't surrendered, their willpower strength is thereby crippled and they can't stick to their diets. Then, because they repeat this scenario time after time, they begin to genuinely doubt their ability to succeed. And finally their doubts become a self-fulfilling prophecy which cannot be broken.

Until now, that is. Now you can start getting your willpower in tip-top shape with the exercises on the following pages. If you've got a problem with decisiveness, turn to the next chapter for some real answers on how to solve that problem.

If your strength of willpower is too wimpy to produce success, flip to Chapter 5 and begin a program to develop this willpower attribute so it's as vibrant and nimble as the others.

Or, you may find that sustaining a continuing desire to stick to your diet is the major stumbling block. You'll find your answers to that problem in Chapter 6.

But don't stop there! Not only should you beef up the willpower attributes that have been letting you down, you also should strengthen *all* your willpower components to give you the best possible chance to make this the last time you ever diet again. In other words, read all of the chapters thoroughly. Then in the final chapter, you'll learn how to put the various willpower-building steps into an organized whole that will make your dieting life infinitely easier and ultimately successful.

Willpower attributes are like links in a chain: the chain is often no stronger than the weakest link. To make sure you're going to be a dieting winner next time, just make sure you've got all your willpower links in tiptop shape. And with that, let's get started. Let's decide to diet, once and for all!

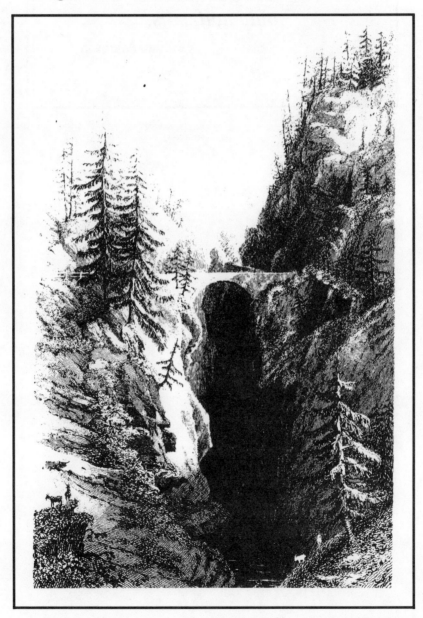

He who fails
only half wills.

—William Atkinson

How to Become a Willing Dieter through Willpower Decisiveness

Give me five minutes with someone who's starting a diet and I'll tell you whether they're going to be successful or not.

Does that sound like unwarranted braggadocio? Well maybe, but I don't think so. While it may seem as if I'm being wildly presumptuous, there are certain key indices which suggest whether a dieter means business or whether he or she is out for another cyclical ride around weight-loss park.

Lest you start thinking that I'm some sort of genius, I'll quickly humble myself by saying that you can do it, too, and just as easily as you see through the excuses proffered by your eight-year-old who claims he didn't take the last three brownies in the cookie jar.

All you have to do is *listen* to what the dieter says. Then carefully sift it through the filter I'm about to give you. Naturally, that's easier to do when you're evaluating someone else's behavior. But you can, with a little honest effort, come clean with yourself, too, and begin your next diet in earnest.

The Revealing Truth

I have interviewed a great many men and women who have successfully quit various unhealthy habits. The differences between the winners and the losers go far beyond mere smoking and nonsmoking, drinking and abstinence, dieting and overeating. And interestingly enough, some of the differences are noticeable even *before* dieters begin their respective journeys to success or failure.

Often I could see their forthcoming success in the way they look, the way they carry themselves, their gestures, their confident smiles. But more importantly, I could hear it in the way they talk. Their very words were reflections of the crucial shift from what psychologists call "compliance vs. surrender."

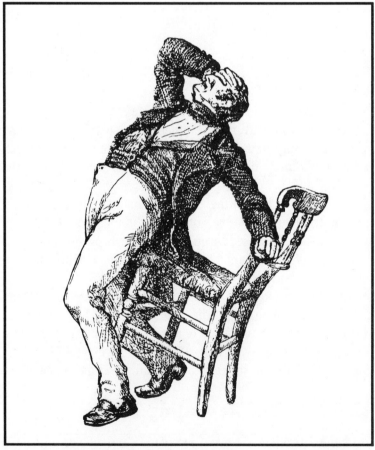

Gaining another pound is serious business for some dieters.

Compliance vs. Surrender

You can "do" a diet in one of two ways. You can *comply* with a diet. Or you can *surrender* to a diet. And they are as different as a wedge of chocolate cake is from a slice of RyKrisp.

Compliant dieting behavior is far more common and a good deal more flimsy than surrender. According to Dr. Harry M. Tiebout who has studied such behavior, compliance is a word that portrays mixed feelings, divided sentiments. Compliance means "agreeing, going along." There is a willingness not to argue or resist, but the cooperation to diet is a bit grudging, a little forced. In short, you may decide to diet, but you're not entirely happy about doing so. You have inner reservations that make your willpower thin and watery.

In my interviews with dieters, these inner reservations become known to me when I asked them the five questions that separate winners from "also rans." And since you are here with me reading this page, I'll ask you the same questions:

1. Why are you overweight?
2. Are you willing to *change* the behavior which makes you overweight?
3. How are you going to do that?
4. When are you going to do that?
5. What are you going to do if and when your plan fails?

Dieters who are going to comply with their diet answer these questions in what I call Dietspeak, those wishy-washy dieting statements that are nothing more than polite rationalizations that reflect the dieter's failure to unify conflicting goals. They were simply trying to put the best face on intentions which belied their very words.

Dieting Commitment or Dietspeak?

Dieters who comply invariably talk to me with statements cobbled with qualifiers such as "maybe," "kind of," "as soon as I can," "I should," "I don't like to," "I might," "I really ought to," "I don't know," "I'll try," "not now," "I suppose I could," etc. All sorts of words and phrases that dilute their willpower and misrepresent their true colors.

Take question number one, for example. Dieters who comply are vague and indifferent to the reasons they're overweight. They somehow believe all of that information will magically appear before their eyes or that Charlton Heston will pay them a housecall with tablets of stone containing the Ten Commandments of Dieting Success.

Or take question two, "Are you willing to give up the behavior(s) that made you overweight in the first place?" Dieters who comply often answer that question with "I think so," or "I'll try," or "maybe."

As if that's not vague enough, compliant dieters know little about *how* they're going to become thin again. That's because they're used to pinning their hopes on the next fad diet, rather than the more important internal prioritizing that must occur before they can become successful with any diet.

"I *think* I might try the XYZ Diet next time. I heard it's very good. I'll *try* it and see what happens."

Or perhaps they'll say, "I know jogging is a great way to burn up calories *but I don't like to jog"* (or alternately, "I'm too busy," or, "I'm afraid of being mugged," or, "the wind will muss my hair").

As to the question of "when" the compliance dieter is going to start, s/he'll say something like, "I'll try to diet *but I'm going to wait because the holiday season is so difficult."* Or, "I want to lose all this weight but *I just don't have time for a regular exercise program."* Or worse yet, "I *really should* go on another diet" (the unannounced inner reservation here is, "but I'm not going to right now").

Here are some more of those compliant statements: "I'll do anything *reasonable* to lose weight." "You know, I *really should* go on a diet."

"I think"? "I'll try"? "I don't like"? Come on, give it up. That kind of talk is cheap and you know as well as I do that it will buy you nothing more than an all-expense-paid dieting guilt trip.

I hope you can see that the compliant dieter is a house divided. These dieters invent all manner of two-faced replies designed to serve two mutually exclusive masters. On the one hand, they try to imply that they're really serious about this dieting business. Conversely, they recognize their own unwillingness or lack of confidence to give their goal undivided support. So they rationalize. They trot out answers which are sufficiently vague to cover any eventuality.

Saying, "I'll *try* to lose weight" sounds a lot like "I *will* lose weight" but it's really quite different. Promising yourself that you'll start a regular exercise program as *soon as you can* is the same sort of semantic doubletalk. These little escape hatches make a dieter's pledge worthless. And that's just as true whether Dietspeak is used out loud, or whether you just think in Dietspeak.

The Enemy Within

What's happening here is that there are really two of you dieting: your conscious and your subconscious. The conscious mind of the compliant dieter says, "I really want to lose all this weight." But his/her subconscious mind is singing a different tune. It says, "Hey, wait a minute. I don't want to change *my* goals. I don't want to diet *now.* I don't want to give up my old eating behavior. I don't want to exercise. But I'll tell you what. I'll go along with your diet for now. But later on it's my turn. I'll let you know when I'm tired of being hungry."

How Dieting Compliance Manifests Itself

Compliant dieters begin diets really believing that they're going all the way because they haven't honestly *listened* to the double messages they deliver with rhetorical guile. When they proclaim to themselves, family and friends that they're honestly "going to try to diet again," they're unaware that Mr. or Ms. Hyde has different ideas.

And thus, lurking surreptitiously just beneath those placid mental waters is the baleful desire to slide back to the old fat ways and all those delicious, fattening foods. The "other dieter," the subconscious, is playing those "old tapes" of past eating behavior *pianissimo,* just out of the conscious' earshot.

But as the diet wears on and the problems of life and the boredom of dieting weaken his or her resolve, those naughty messages begin to seep into the chinks of his or her dieting armor.

From seemingly out of nowhere those mischievous little ideas start oozing into conscious thought. Like bat-winged phantoms they inexplicably surface before one's mental eyes—shameful desires clothed in the sheepskin of "rational" thought.

You've heard them before. Sentences like, "I've been good. I'll just eat this one little treat. I can handle it." Or, "I'm pretty busy today. I'll try to do my exercise routine later. Besides, I've lost a lot of weight already. One day won't hurt." Or "I'll cheat today but I'll get back on my diet tomorrow."

Strength of willpower can handle just so many of these satanic assaults from the subconscious, but not all. And that's the point. Given enough of these sentences, the compliant dieter starts obeying those suggestions from down below. First he snitches a cookie. Then, a candy bar. Next he's buying a pint of ice cream.

And as inevitably as ants on picnic Sundays, when your diet starts falling apart, so does your exercise program (I mean, why exercise when you're not on a diet?). Then it's right back into all the old behavior that your subconscious wanted all along: Lots of eating. Lots of laziness. Lots of fat. Lots of guilt. And it keeps bulding until one hellish day when it weighs so heavily on your mind and body that your conscience guiltily decides that it's "diet time" again.

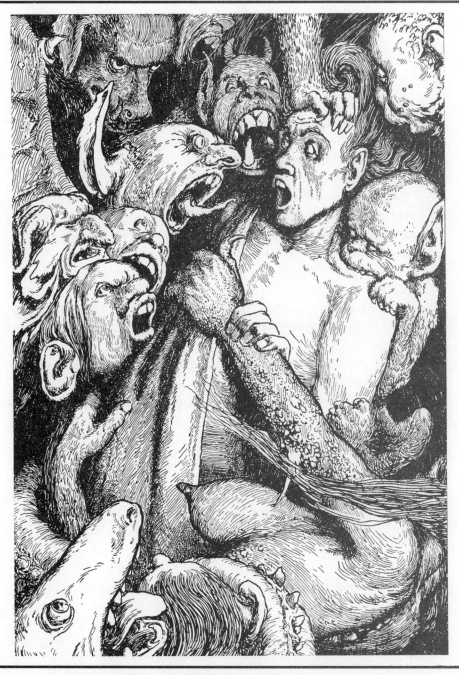

Anytime you diet, quiet little voices will sometimes urge you to engage in a little cheating.

Surrender

Surrender is something entirely different. And that's because the messages borne by both the conscious and the subconscious mind are one and the same! There is no inner division.

Surrender means enthusiastic, wholehearted and complete agreement to diet, once and for all. There's nothing wishy-washy about this willpower decision: the dieter is unequivocal, sincere and honest.

Having made this shift, it's as if the dieter has entered a new force field and the filings of willpower have lined up in a convincing new formation. The result is that the willpower now has an eye more for possibilities than impediments.

When she talks her choice of words is substantially different from the compliant dieter. Her decision to diet is anchored in terms that are precise and forthright. Her language contains no hidden meanings. No trap doors. No escape hatches. No fine print.

She uses phrases like, "I'm going to get rid of this fat, right now, once and for all."

"I'm overweight because I graze on high-calorie snacks in front of the TV all night and I don't get regular exercise and I'm going to put an end to that right now."

"I am going on the XYZ diet starting today."

"If I goof, I'll start over. Right now."

"I've made up my mind and I can do it."

"I'm going to start jogging."

"I'm beginning today."

"I will."

"Now!"

When the dieter unshackles her willpower by removing the chains of precondition, she is frequently catapulted to instant victory. She has *already* won the weight-loss battle. Losing weight is a mere caloric formality since her willpower will freely and automatically invoke the psychological forces that she previously believed were unnecessary.

Still unconvinced? Then listen to the way these successful

dieters talked after they made the shift from compliance to surrender and compare it to your own thinking:

Janice, who went from 215 to 124 pounds said: "Everything I knew about dieting was already in my head. I had been on lots of diets and knew the calorie counts of everything from dry toast to pizza. Anyway, one day I stepped on the scale and I was just mortified to find that I had gained seven pounds since the first of the week. And I was supposed to be dieting. I sat down and cried. Then I got mad. I hated myself. And I hated my diet.

"I don't know why but at that moment, things just suddenly clicked. Everything made sense for me. It all came together. I could see that I had been just sliding by on my previous diets and wasn't about to stick to them. I was just fooling myself. Now I was ready to win."

A forty-six-year-old electrician told me: "One day I was lying on my couch at home watching the TV and I looked at myself and was thoroughly disgusted. I said to myself, 'Frank, you are a fat slob.' I was eating something at the time and I put it down. And that was that. I started a diet right that moment and I haven't been fat since."

Sue, thirty-two, went from 210 to 133 pounds. She said her weight had ballooned to 195 pounds when she had her last child. "I felt so miserable being fat that I made a promise not to ever get that heavy again. But it wasn't long after that when I hit 210 and I weighed more than my husband. A lot more! When I saw those numbers on the scale it hit me like a ton of bricks. 'What the hell is going on here?' I asked myself. And I spent the whole day thinking about what a failure I was. About all the diets I had tried and failed. I knew very well what I had been doing. I had been just playing games with myself. I hadn't really settled down. Well, I did settle down and I haven't been fat since."

Virginia was in her mid-thirties and had been overweight for nearly ten years. Her body had blossomed with about thirty excess pounds, which, when stacked on her 5'2" frame, distended her otherwise pleasant features.

"I have done practically every diet that ever existed," she told me. "Sometimes I'd quit my diet when I got close to my ideal weight. Other times I'd get upset about something and break down long before I got my weight down.

"But one day after I had just finished booting my umpteenth diet I seemed to feel different. I was really down on myself. You know, I had really been working on this diet. I mean, I had really tried. But still I failed. I felt so hopeless.

"Suddenly I realized that this was a no-win situation. I just couldn't go on doing this dieting business only to fail again and again. I had to put a stop to it all.

"That's when I began to think differently.

"I began to realize that I had really been kidding myself. Every time I started a diet I was secretly waiting for the time when I could start eating again. And not just eating. I mean eating all those things that would make me fat again. I just hadn't accepted the fact that I had to change; that change was the only way out.

"My logical mind accepted all those reasons for wanting to be thin, but deep down inside I was just as unaccepting as ever. Once I realized that I had been conning myself, I knew I could make it. I didn't quit—I surrendered."

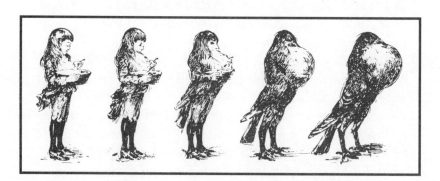

How to Surrender

The dieters whose experiences I have just shared reached their decision to surrender to their diet in a rather intuitive fashion. That is, they used their heart instead of their head. Psychologists refer to this phenomenon as "intuition." It's the spontaneous knowing of something without the conscious use of understanding. You might say it's the ability to perceive the "big picture" without conscious reasoning or thinking about it.

It's like the old comic strip visual of the lightbulb over the character's head. But while you might think the bulb lit in one, blinding flash, it had, in fact, been warming up a long time. In fact, what usually happens is that a cumulative series of events builds until one precipitous day, some dramatic event presents reality to them in such a cold, heartless way that surrender for them becomes inescapable.

Your doctor warns you about the impending consequences of your excess fat.

Your closest friend succeeds in losing weight while you remain as fat as ever.

Your weight hits an all-time high as your spirits hit an all-time low.

Someone at a party asks when the baby is due and you're not pregnant.

Your lover turns another chilly backside to your nocturnal advance.

Victory by Surrender

Dramatic situations like these can trigger dieters into *instant* surrender to dieting realities. Again and again successful dieters told me that "something clicked," and from then on they had the willpower to succeed. Dieting became almost easy *because they began to invoke their full complement of willpower skills and attributes.* Vagueness and indifference have been cast aside. Where they were once passengers, they now were captains of their fate.

William James, dean of American psychologists, cites example after example of people who have tried unsuccessfully to rid themselves of bad habits only to find that success came when they surrendered, when they gave up the conscious struggle and allowed their willpower to do its duty naturally, effortlessly.

Interestingly enough, most dieters find it is only after having "seen the light" that they finally realized the previous snow job they had been giving themselves. They began to understand that all the worry, stress, and strain of their previous dieting attempts was absolutely useless. That the real way to achieve success is to let go and let your willpower do whatever is necessary to accomplish its purpose.

But that's hardly consolation to those who haven't surrendered. And unless you want to gain a hundred more pounds so you get truly sick of yourself, or find yourself a lover who can subsequently give you the cold shoulder, you're really back at square one again.

The Five Steps of Surrender

It's not an easy matter to surrender. Many times dieters have told me that they thought they had surrendered, only to find out later that they hadn't. It's obvious our minds can do a pretty good job of fooling ourselves.

But it can be done. And I have found that the most effective means of getting dieters to surrender is to give them a better picture of the thinking that goes on in the minds of dieters who have, in fact, successfully surrendered. When you have a clear-cut target to shoot for, you'll have a course to follow and signposts to lead you.

Successful dieters have told me there are five unmistakable signs along their road from compliance to surrender. They have finally agreed, both consciously and subconsciously, that:

1. Being fat is my number one problem
2. There's only *one* solution

3. The problem won't go away

4. *I* am responsible for solving the problem

5. I'll gladly do *anything* necessary to become thin

1. Being Fat Is My Number One Problem

The first major change that surrender produces is a major shifting in priorities. The problem of being overweight is deliberately moved to the front burner. The dieter may have other problems or ambitions in his or her life, but the Number One problem is losing weight. All other goals and activities are assembled around the diet, rather than the other way around. And he refuses to allow his subconscious to arrange his life in such a way as to prevent him from reaching his goal.

Case in point. Many dieters complain that they don't have time to do a regular exercise program. What they really mean is they don't always have a convenient time to do their exercises.

But, if you've really surrendered to the dictum that you *must* exercise regularly to lose and maintain weight, your perception of the problem changes. The exercise program becomes the "given," the variable becomes the rest of your daily activity. By that I mean you'll fit your life into your exercise program, rather than your exercise program into your life. And you'll do it *willingly*.

You'll get up an hour early to do your exercises. You'll go to bed an hour later. You'll do exercises on your lunch hour and eat when (and if) you have the chance. And when Mary calls and says "Let's have lunch Thursday," you'll say, "I'm sorry, but I exercise at noon. How about 1:30?" But you won't allow yourself to say, "I don't have time" to do exercises. You'll find a way, or make a way to do it, even though that means reordering your present life-style.

2. The Situation Is Hopeless— There's Only One Way Out

The artful dodge is over. You have run out of excuses. Acts of denial are useless prevarications. You have finally realized that the dieting prognosis is absolutely immutable: You cannot get slim unless you *stay* on a diet and *stick* to an exercise program as well. There are absolutely no other alternatives. No ifs, no maybes, no buts. *You must stick to your diet.*

Many dieters spend life in some sort of never-never land where all things seem possible. They believe, for example, that they can stay thin, but allow themselves all sorts of high-calorie treats as well. Sorry. In dieting as in life, you get what you pay for. There are no free rides. If you want to run the Boston Marathon, you have to accept the fact that you've got to train heavily to do it. Running two or three times a week just won't cut it. If you want to be a concert pianist, it will never suffice to practice only when you feel like it. And if you want to lose weight and stay slim forever, you know the price you've got to pay: diet and exercise. It's that simple.

3. The Problem Won't Go Away

Like an elephant in your bedroom, being overweight is a problem that just won't go away. Dieters who have surrendered tell me this truism is now given honest recognition. Excess fat cannot be wished away. Nor can you, with all due respect, pray it away.

I remember recognizing this signpost myself and the mental fork in the road it represented. The good news was I recognized in myself a remarkably strong degree of persistence. I deeply wanted to rid myself of a thirty-pound doughnut of fat that had congealed around my waist. And I knew I would persist, forever if need be, to do it.

The bad news was that I also was unwilling to let go of the old eating behavior that kept me in varying degrees of overweightness all the time. It was a no-win situation. I could not travel both pathways at once. I had to make a decision. Either I'd have to forget my goal of getting thin (which I couldn't), or I'd have to let go of my old, overeating behavior which I could do, but was reluctant. Once I identified and *accepted* the incompatibility of my thinking, surrender came easily.

4. *I* Am Responsible for Solving the Problem

That's when dieters who have surrendered face up to the inevitable: *I* am responsible for getting myself thin. Yes, it would be nice to get some help from family, friends, or dieting experts, but don't count on it. It's your problem. And it's not up to them to solve it.

"No food plan is going to work for you unless you are willing to give up your old body," said Richard Simmons. "When you make up your mind to get on a sensible food plan and a healthful exercise program and stick to them until you reach your goal, you can accomplish anything."

Dieters who have surrendered not only understand the truth of this statement. They *accept* it.

5. I'll Gladly Do *Whatever* I Must to Become Thin

The fifth and final principle of surrender is tractability. Dieters who have surrendered and assumed responsibility for their overweightness became very honest and *eager* to find ways to stick to their dieting and exercising programs.

No, not the begrudging kind of dieting. Not a reluctant "going along." Not the resentful sort of compliance that used to accompany declarations such as: "I just can't have that hunk of apple pie; I'm on a diet." Not the half-hearted disdain for sweets and snacks while just beneath the surface smolders a burning desire to covet them.

Gandhi said it better than anyone. "Dietary restrictions undertaken by those who lust after food have no effect. They keep their bodies without food, but feast their minds on all sorts of delicacies, thinking all the while what they will eat and drink after their diet is over." (And you thought I was kidding when I said Gandhi had written a diet book.)

The winners are different. They showed instead a whole-hearted and *sincere* acceptance that those sinful treats are nice, but being thin is even nicer. More than an acceptance that they cannot have it both ways, they made a positive affirmation to find a way, or make a way to stick to their diets. To which I offer the following truism to hang on your refrigerator door:

If your diet is a continual struggle, you probably haven't surrendered. Dieters who eventually win the weight-loss battle will tell you they won only after it no longer was a battle.

Finding Personal Solutions

It's this final step that motivates dieters to look for their own personal solutions to their dieting dilemma. One sure

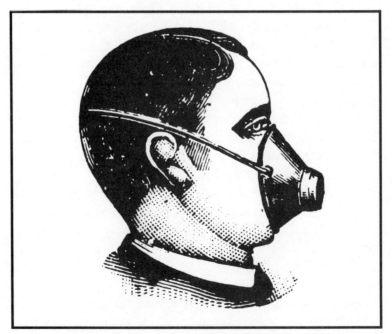

Most dieters find personal solutions to stick to their diet.

sign that you've surrendered is when you start to do the same.

So it was that I found out about the B. Dalton Green Bean Diet. I shouldn't wonder if you haven't heard about it. I gave it that name because I learned of it while signing autographs at a suburban Minneapolis B. Dalton Bookseller.

Unless your name is something like Jane Fonda or Mike Wallace, bookstore autograph signings can be low-key affairs with short lines of dedicated fans flanked by other customers who think you're somebody famous like Leo Buscaglia or maybe some other celebrity they'd like to hug.

Although I am distinctly huggable but hardly famous, my autograph signings tend to be quiet exercises in penmanship, occasioned by a few people who actually want to buy my book or comment on its subject.

It was during one of these quiet spells that a woman approached me, not to buy my dieting book, but to tell me about her diet. She told me she had lost nearly fifty pounds dieting on green beans. Green beans for breakfast. Beans for lunch. Beans for dinner.

"Why green beans?" I asked.

"Well, I heard that beans were real low in calories so I decided to keep myself filled with them."

Obviously, this is the kind of diet against which doctors and nutritionists uniformly inveigh. A diet as nutritionally balanced as Mary Lou Retton and William "Refrigerator" Perry on a teeter-totter. But it's the diet that worked for this woman, and believe it or not, many other dieters have told me they successfully use the Green Bean Diet, too.

Successful Dieters
Do It Their Own Way

Since the Green Bean Diet has worked for so many dieters, shouldn't I recommend it to others? I mean, if it worked for them, couldn't it work for you?

Probably not.

Why? Because it's not *your* solution. It would offer you

about as much help as those dieting tips which garnish the pages of women's magazines and newspaper family sections.

Successful dieters have told me they can occasionally use these paltry morsels of authoritative wisdom. But far more beneficial are the tips they invent for themselves. As I've said, it's a sure sign that you have surrendered to your diet when you begin to search for these personalized strokes of dieting genius. These activities are vivid evidence that you're deadly serious about finding the answers to your overweight problem.

Have You Surrendered?

As your first exercise in building winning willpower, I want you to take an inventory of your dieting life to discover whether you've truly surrendered to your diet. Think about what you've read and how these steps apply to your dieting life. Make a vigorous and painstaking effort to discover where you are on the continuum from compliance to surrender. Have you surrendered to some of the principles but not others? Have you finally made the decision to accept the diet and win the weight-loss battle?

This first exercise attempts to put before your eyes, solid, realistic evidence of whether you've surrendered to your diet; whether you've unleashed your complete willpower. And more importantly, it will open your mental eyes so you can make the shift and win with your next diet.

It's a smart idea to write down your answers to the steps. Isolate and identify the evidence which supports your belief you have surrendered to the five principles. Find examples that demonstrate your compliance. Perhaps you have stubbornly clung to the eating behavior which has gotten you in trouble time after time. Are you now willing to give up this behavior? What evidence do you have to support that belief?

What it boils down to is this: If you aren't willing to give up the behavior which got you fat in the first place, why go on another diet?

Your Surrender vs. Compliance Inventory

1. Is being fat your number one problem?

Do you refuse to reorder your priorities to accomplish the dieting goal? What sort of compromises are you willing to accept? Are you rearranging your life in such a way that dieting is number one?

2. Do you think your fat body will miraculously "fade away?"

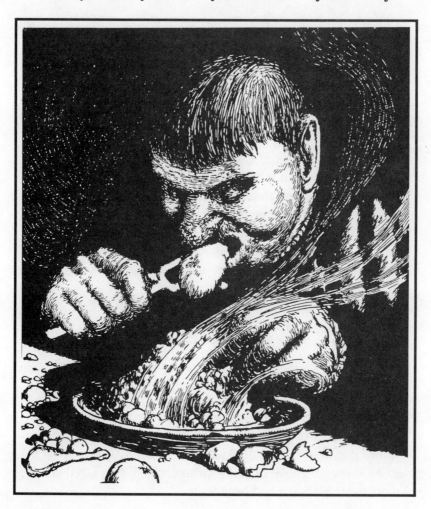

Are you waiting for the miracle pill to be invented that allows you to eat anything you want and still maintain a slim figure? Are you pinning your weight-loss hopes on the next fad diet?

3. Do you believe there's more than one solution to the dieting dilemma?

Are you a special case? Can you repeal the laws of dieting to such a degree that you can stay slim without exercising? Without regulating your diet?

4. Who's responsible for solving your overweight problem?

Are you blaming your overweightness on somebody else? On diets that "don't work"? On family, friends, spouse, or lover who fail to support your dieting effort?

Are you hiding behind some physical problem which you think is responsible for your overweightness?

5. Will you do *anything* necessary to become thin?

No, I don't mean you'll climb Mt. Everest or run a marathon. I mean the actions which are necessary to your dieting success. What's necessary here is that you identify the pre-conditions you place on dieting success and decide what, if anything, you are willing to do about them.

The first part is fairly easy. Just fill in the blanks:

I want to lose weight but I am unwilling to _____,

_____, _____ and _____.

In my own personal life, it used to be that I was unwilling to: (1) give up sugar; (2) give up sodas; (3) give up snacking between 6:00 P.M. and 10:00 P.M. When I made my unequivocal decision to lose weight for good, these are the only questions I had to worry about. And when I finally answered "yes" to all three, my days of being an undecided, two-faced dieter were over. Freedom had been won.

Now, how about you? What preconditions have you established? Will you do the exercises in this book? Will you read other books? WIll you keep a dieting diary? Will you give up sugar? Will you stick to a regular program of exercise? What aren't you willing to do? And more important, is there a yawning gap between what you're *willing* to do and what you *have to do* to lose weight for good? And if there is, what are you going to do about it?

All Things Are Possible

As you meditate on the problems of compliant dieting behavior, you'll begin to see the incompatibilities of your past dieting behavior. You'll begin to "see the light," just as the other successful dieters did. You'll agree that successful dieting is, indeed, a state of mind, not a physical condition.

Famous psychologist Dr. Albert Ellis, author of the bestselling *Guide to Rational Living* and a number of other critically acclaimed self-help books, agrees. Ellis, writing in the *British Journal of Cognitive Psychotherapy*, says anyone who is prepared to work to reach his weight-loss goal can do so, if he reconciles his "irrational beliefs" that he can lose weight and eat anything he wants.

When this reconciliation in thinking occurs, surrender occurs, and dieting success becomes possible. The dieter will now use her willpower to do whatever is necessary to become thin. Food plans that previously were viewed as too restrictive become tolerable. Extra planning to avoid holiday bingeing is cheerfully, eagerly anticipated as the alternative to overeating and spending more grueling months on the dieting treadmill. A regular program of exercise that was previously neglected because it was (pick your excuse) too expensive, too time-consuming, or too hard, will now, on average, become enjoyable.

The "new dieter" warmly welcomes these components into her repertoire of weight-loss techniques and she jealously guards against any infringement on her plan. Having found shoes that fit, she steps into them and walks with a new confidence. She has done a complete about-face. The change is remarkable, complete, and it is, above all else, the key to her eventual success.

Getting to Yes

Dieting success can now be your success, if you can make the crucial shift from compliance to surrender. The trouble is, though, I can talk to you until I'm blue in the face and I can't make you surrender to your diet. It has to come from within you.

I'm sorry about that. I know I'm beginning to sound like the magazine articles on dieting, but it's true. "I can talk to you till I'm old and shrunken," says Richard Simmons, "but none of this will make a difference. The weight loss has to be your need and the discipline has to come from within you."

Keep Thinking, Keep Trying

But I believe that you can pave the way for your surrender by continuing to reread this chapter and reflect again and again on these five questions. And that's what I want you to do. Read it every day until you can answer "yes" to every question. Wholeheartedly. Completely. Honestly.

Once you've made the decision to undertake your next diet "no holds barred," I know you'll be a winner with the help of the remaining exercises in this book.

It is will,
force of purpose,
that enables a man
to do or be whatever
he sets his mind on
being or doing.

—William W. Atkinson

Six Exercises to Build Willpower Strength

There are those times in the life of every dieter, every man or woman who wants to lose weight and stay thin. You come face to face with temptation: the crushing urge to snitch some forbidden pleasure loaded with so many calories it's exchangeable for something like two million carrot sticks or one year of hard labor on a Siberian salt pile.

You may be simply dying for a plateful of brownies. You may want a pizza pie so bad you can taste it. Everything painful about hunger and cravings has been rolled up into one unmerciful ball that is hurtling down your path to dieting freedom as if you were playing the lead in *Indiana Jones and the Temple of Dieting*.

At that point, whether the temptation is a razor-thin instant or agonizing minutes or hours, we confront head-on the decision of whether to continue our diet or give in to caloric enticement. On the one hand we have our deep desire to lose weight and become thin again. And on the other, we have food about us everywhere which is just *begging* to be eaten.

It's a true dilemma. We are being forced to choose between two causes of action which, in the blur of hungers both psychic and physiological, both real and imagined, seem precisely of equal value.

The resulting warfare between the forces of dieting good

and evil can invariably be boiled down into this question: Are you going to let this amorphous enemy seize the moment and send your diet into a temporary stall? And if you do, will this little white dieting slip signal the beginning of a backslide of such bingeful proportions that you'll never recover?

Or, optimistically, will the strength of your willpower grasp the slender thread of dieting sanity and raise you to higher, safer ground?

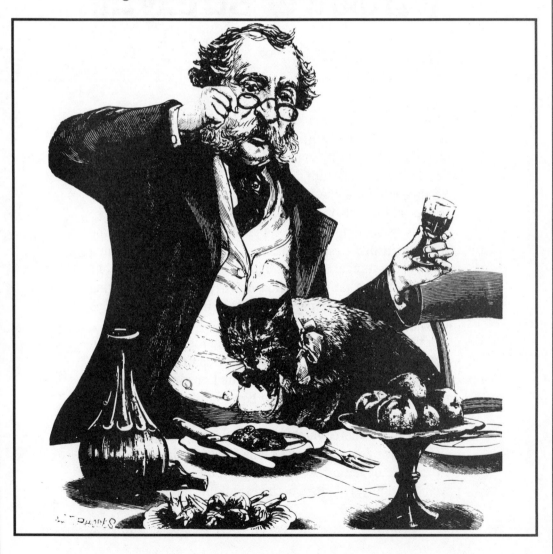

Willpower and Changing Behavior

All major changes of behavior can be reduced to a series of little do or diet scenarios such as this, occasions when we seem to be drawn to forbidden foods with the gravitational pull of a celestial black hole. And many dieters think this is exactly what dieting is all about: those times when absolutely nothing stands between them and cheating except the sheer, naked, glorious strength of willpower.

When we start a diet, we are likely to be confronted by many enemies which are capable of defeating our dieting plans. But as you know, when new behavior gradually takes root in habit, the occasions for decisions like this generally become fewer and fewer. The trick, then, is to get from point A to point B with enough frequency so as to build a reservoir of successful performance.

For example, the nonsmoking tenderfoot in the beginning will think about, and argue with, himself about whether to have a cigarette twenty or thirty times a day. More often than not, he or she will use strength of will to refrain from having the cigarette and begin to build the foundation for a healthy new habit.

The following week, these occasions may fall to just five or ten. Using the added strength their past successes have given them, they become better able to fend off these cravings. The occasions for these smoking snares become fewer and fewer in the weeks and months that follow. Finally, there comes a time when it isn't an issue at all. They just never think of smoking.

Athletic Willpower

Athletes know this better than anyone. They must spend countless lonely hours honing their skills in hopes of winning eventual victory. The great marathoner Grete Waitz is an example. Waitz has a record of marathon victories which is the envy of millions. But she has a training schedule which would give most of us second thoughts about becoming a world-class marathoner.

Not only does Grete run seven days a week, but most days, she runs twice! When she's in training, Waitz says she rarely thinks about not running, so deeply ingrained is her running habit.

But Grete isn't alone in her devotion to daily running. The jogging world is full of all kinds of resolute runners whose running feats far surpass anything Grete does even though they're recreational runners: runners who log twenty or thirty miles a day; runners who perform in marathons not once or twice a year like Waitz, but once a week. Still others have set records for the number of consecutive days they've run, often two or three years of steady running, day in and day out, without missing a day.

Habits like that can be formed with surprising ease if you *will* to do so. You start out small, build, and sooner or later a new, healthier habit is born to guide your future.

The key here is that it becomes easier the more often you do your thing. And within four to eight weeks, most new behavior begins to take the form of habit.

The same thing is true of building strength of willpower. If you say "no" enough times, it will become habit. After that, you won't even have to think about it. You won't have to discuss it. The answer will already have been made. No argument. No dissent. Just the desirable action.

Developing a Strong Will

Many exercises have been developed to help you build the strength of willpower that can help you say "no" (or alternately, "yes") enough times so you can stick to your diet and stay slim as long as you like. These exercises are built on the premise that we build willpower when we ask it to perform activities primarily for the purpose of building willpower alone.

Too often in life we develop a tried and proven routine to which we stick with monotonous regularity. In our rutted existences, we use about 1 percent willpower; 99 percent habit. We get up at the same time. Put on the same sort of clothes. We eat the same breakfasts. Take the same route to work and upon arrival, we spend eight hours doing pretty much the same thing. Next we take the same route home, eat variations on about a half-dozen or so different meals, watch the same TV shows each night before we get up the next day to repeat the whole boring tableau over again.

There's not a whole lot of call for willpower here. And willpower strength which continues to sit on the bench of life grows flaccid from disuse. When called upon to perform feats requiring considerable discipline, particularly those that require you to go head-to-head with some instinctual craving like smoking, eating, alcohol, or drugs, willpower strength often fails miserably.

These exercises are designed to take you out of your rutted existence and put you in the driver's seat. You're your own boss. You run the show. They are designed to increase your ability to *do what you don't want to do*. And when your willpower can do that in non-dieting behavior, it can do so in dieting behavior.

SIX EXERCISES THAT BUILD WILLPOWER STRENGTH

1. Doing the disagreeable
2. Doing it now
3. Doing it later
4. Doing the "useless"
5. Doing it your way
6. Acting as if

1. Doing the Disagreeable

"Nothing schools the will and renders it ready for effort in this complex world better than accustoming it to face disagreeable things," said Halleck. "The only way to secure such a will is to practice doing disagreeable things."

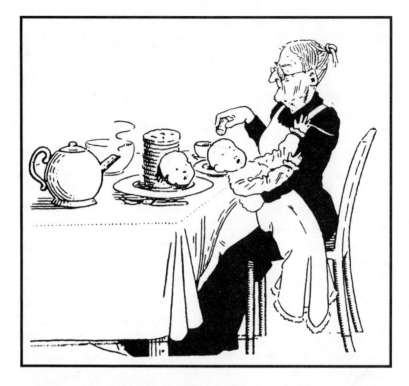

The dieter who habitually avoids disagreeable action is training his willpower to be useless at a time when supreme effort is demanded. When push comes to caloric shove, your goal is to say "No thanks" with enough regularity that you stick to your diet.

Starting today, I want you to begin doing the disagreeable. Look for the things in your life which you don't like to do, and *do* them. There are probably hundreds you could choose from, but since they're personal to your life, I can't choose them for you.

Keep in mind, they will have nothing to do with dieting. But they're needed to help build the strength of will you need to diet successfully. Each time you find a disagreeable task to perform, remind yourself of why you're doing it: "I am going to clean the bathroom because I want to build willpower!"

By doing tasks of this sort, you will not only strengthen your willpower, but also serve notice to yourself that you can, in fact, do whatever you will to do. You may even say so out loud. "As an exercise to strengthen my willpower, I am going to clean the bathroom (or whatever it is you promise to do). I know this is something I dislike doing, and that is precisely why I am doing it."

Repeating these kinds of activities inculcates upon your mind that you are in charge of your destiny—not luck, not fear, not chance circumstance, nor exterior event.

Here are a few exercises that students of my willpower classes have told me they have done with good results.

1. Regularly taking the garbage out
2. Balancing the checkbook
3. Answering correspondence
4. Writing "thank you" notes promptly
5. Washing the bathroom floor
6. Washing dishes
7. Mowing the lawn
8. Washing windows
9. Grocery shopping
10. Cleaning up after the dog
11. Calling the in-laws
12. Meal planning
13. Getting a haircut
14. Doing tax work
15. Exercising
16. Cleaning the bathtub
17. Cleaning house
18. Washing clothes
19. Shaving their legs
20. Going to the dentist
21. Driving behind a slow-moving truck

2. Doing It Now

The second exercise to help you build strength of will is doing ordinary tasks *right now*. Do not put off until tomorrow what you can do today.

In his bestseller, *Stop Procrastinating—Do It*, author Dr.

James R. Sherman has chronicled the many reasons why people get in the habit (there's that word again) of procrastinating and he shows how to stop this harmful habit. One of Sherman's suggestions is to practice doing small things *right now*. Instead of waiting, as you usually do, start small and do it now.

Again, as part of this exercise, *tell yourself* why you're doing the exercise. Tell yourself, for example, "Just as an exercise to build my willpower, I am going to answer all my correspondence the moment I receive it." Or, "Just for today to build my willpower, I will wash the dishes immediately after dinner and not wait until later."

Whatever you would prefer to put off, make a point starting today to do it now! Make sure you tell yourself that you're doing it as a willpower building exercise. You'll be surprised how soon you'll be using your strong willpower to control your dieting life just as successfully.

3. Doing It Later

Another exercise which students of willpower find very effective, except a little more difficult to do, is "doing it later." By that I mean, select several things you *like* to do but postpone action.

If you like to read the newspaper first thing in the morning, put it off—as an exercise to build your strength of willpower—until sometime later in the day.

Perhaps you like to watch TV. Fine, instead of starting at 7 P.M., start at 8 P.M. If you like to eat lunch at noon, settle for 2 P.M. The lunch hour crowds will be that much thinner.

Used to opening your mail as soon as you get to the office or home? Do it when you come back from that new luncheon spot or the following morning.

Like to answer your telephone messages as soon as you receive them? Put if off until later.

You get the idea. Doing these exercises not only builds your strength of willpower, but helps you run your life any way you want. You just have to be *willing* to do so.

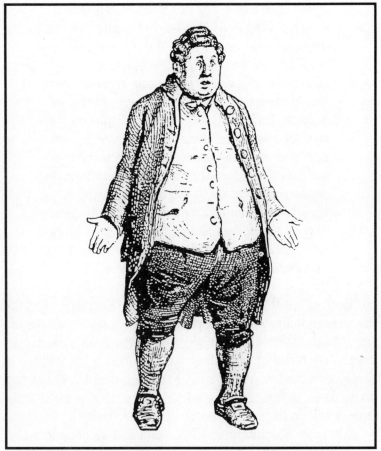

"I had no idea I was eating nine thousand calories a day!"

4. Doing the Useless

This sort of activity is like that first proposed by psychologist and philosopher William James. Here is what James said:

> *Keep alive in yourself the faculty of making efforts by means of little useless exercises every day. That is to say, be systematically heroic every day in little unnecessary things; do something every other day for the sole and simple reason that it is difficult and you would prefer not to do it, so that when the cruel hour of danger*

strikes, you will not be unnerved or unprepared. A self-discipline of this kind is similar to the insurance that one pays on one's house and on one's possessions. To pay the premium is not pleasant and possibly may never serve us, but should it happen that our house were burnt, the payment will save us from ruin. Similarly, the man who has accustomed himself steadily, for day after day, to concentrate his attention, to will his energy, for instance, not to spend money on unnecessary things, will be well rewarded by his effort. When disasters occur, he will stand firm as a rock even though faced on all sides by ruin while his companions in distress will be swept aside as the chaff from the sieve.

"Useless" exercises are abundant. Boyd Barrett, one of the pioneers in willpower development, made himself this resolution: "Each day for the next seven days, I will stand on a chair here in my room for ten consecutive minutes and I will try to do so contentedly. At the end of this ten-minute task, I will write down the mental states I have experienced during that time. I will do the same on each of the seven days."

This is an absolutely terrific exercise. I've done it many, many times myself, both standing on a chair and face-forward into a corner.

This latter exercise I learned about many years ago when a certain plumpish, gray-haired teacher made me stand in the corner. "Charles," she would say, peering through sepia-tinted bifocals so dark they were practically sunglasses, "Charles, will you take up your position in the corner until you learn to behave like the rest of the class?"

It was not a question, of course, it was a command performance. And it was one she made with enough frequency that the whole class knew what "my position" in the corner was.

Mrs. Pettit knew that my little sojourns to the corner of her third-grade classroom of old Warrington elementary school in

Minneapolis somehow refreshed my will to behave myself in her class.

And do you know, she was right. For reasons I never understood at the time, I was able to collect my thoughts during those quiet interludes and soon return to full class participation. Mrs. Pettit has undoubtedly gone to that great schoolroom in the sky never fully knowing what a favor she did to the weary willpower of that little third grader.

The purpose of an exercise like this, of course, is to put yourself in an *unaccustomed* position on purpose; to give yourself "think time" about your willpower and your ability to use it at will. And whether you stand on a chair or in the corner or lean against a table or wall, the result is the same.

Each time you perform an exercise like this, you'll feel within yourself a growing power and ability to flex your willpower muscles. Said Barrett: "This exercise 'tones me up' morally, and awakens in me a sense of nobility and virility. I maintain an attitude not of submission and resignation, but of willing actively what I am doing, and it is this that gives me satisfaction."

When I do this exercise, and willpower students concur, I come in conscious contact with my willpower. In a matter of minutes, as you reflect on your willpower and your ability to do your bidding, you can actually feel your willpower welling up inside your body. This is one of the most effective exercises you can do to build strength of willpower. But it's not the only one.

Barrett had other exercises of the same "useless" type you can try:

1. Repeat quietly and aloud: "*I will* do *this*," keeping time with ryhthmic movements of a stick or ruler for five minutes.

2. Walk to and fro in a room, touching in turn, say, a clock on the mantelpiece and a particular pane of glass for five minutes.

3. Listen to the ticking of a clock or watch (Barrett was writing nearly one hundred years ago) making some definite movements at every fifth tick.

Here are some other useless exercises you can try:

4. Take a handful of paper clips and arrange them on your desk in some irrelevant pattern.

5. Count the grains of sugar from a teaspoon (use a tablespoon if you're brave).

6. Count telephone poles from home to office.

7. Circle the number of times this book uses the word, "willpower." (I've done it, but it wouldn't be fair to tell you.)

8. Take an inventory of all the books in your home or office.

9. Count the number of loops in a square inch of your carpeting.

5. Doing It *Your* Way

This willpower building tool is designed to set you free from the ordinary, the routine, to free you from the rut of life and make you the free spirit on this Earth which you really are.

Starting today, begin doing more things your way. If you take the same route to work, try another. If you eat at the same restaurants, try new ones. If you put your leg into the left leg of your pants first, do it the other way around. If you put on your contact lens after taking a shower, put them on before.

And so on.

One "do it your way" exercise which I sometimes perform when driving my car is to leave the freeway and drive instead on residential streets to reach my downtown office. Granted, it's more inconvenient and markedly slower to drive city streets, but I get an entirely new view of the city while exercising my willpower in a productive new way.

At other times, I am struck by some oddity as I drive along. Impatience and habit usually implore me to ignore the item. But exercising my strength of will, I break my routine, drive around the block, and give the peculiarity second notice.

Yes, it takes extra time. And it occasionally makes me late. But it's my way of reaffirming to myself that *I'm* in charge, and if I want to be late, then I'll *be* late.

Still another exercise I think is an excellent strength builder is purposefully driving behind a slow-moving truck on the freeway. It takes considerable patience and strength of will to do it. But with practice you'll be surprised at how easily you can train yourself to do most *anything* you want.

Each time I will these acts, I realize that I have the willpower to drive my car in any direction I want, or not to drive at all. I am not a creature of habit whose rutted existence is controlled by chance, circumstance, or by others. *I* can at any time choose to do or not do.

And here's another note. Some willpower students have told me that they are already rather independent souls who are used to doing things their own way, or doing things which are disagreeable.

That's fine. But the purpose of the exercise is to build willpower. And that requires us to do things we are not inclined to do. Therefore, if you *like* doing different things all the time, the exercise is unlikely to be a rewarding one for you. Better you should find monotonous things to do.

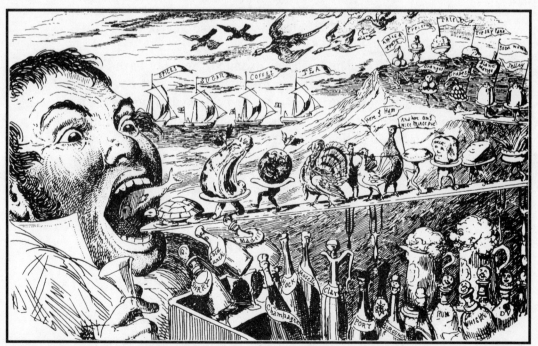

Some dieters use a trifling dieting slip as the occasion for a whole-hog dieting backslide.

I suppose you could say it's the same difference as painting a house, and painting a house because it needs it. You can well imagine that painting a house that doesn't need painting is strictly an exercise of will, not of necessity. Walking around the block six times to build willpower is totally different from walking about the block a haf-dozen times to find your lost son or daughter. See what I mean?

6. Act as if

Finally, there's still another technique for building strength of willpower: simply doing things "as if" you had strong willpower.

The "act as if" formula has been clearly explained in many psychology self-help books going back at least a hundred years. The technique is effective because, although your willpower exerts very little direct control over your emotions and feelings, it still can exert considerable control over your mood. And just as willpower better controls your behavior through the "indirect method," so too can your emotions be controlled better by indirect activity.

When you're depressed, for example, you may have little direct control over your depression, but you still have the power to direct external actions. And when willpower is used to *purposefully* control external actions, it can, indeed, influence *internal* feelings. "Refuse to express a passion," says William James, "and it dies."

> *Count ten before venting your anger and its occasion seems ridiculous. Whistling to keep up courage is no mere figure of speech. On the other hand, sit all day in a moping posture, and reply to everything with a dismal voice and your melancholy lingers. There is no more valuable precept in moral education than this, as all who have experience know: If we wish to conquer undesirable emotional tendencies in ourselves, we must assiduously and in the first instance*

cold-bloodedly go through the posture outward movements of those contrary dispositions which we prefer to cultivate. Smooth the brow, brighten the eye, contract the dorsal rather than the ventral aspect of the frame, and speak in a major key, pass the genial compliment, and your heart must be frigid indeed if it does not gradually thaw.

This exercise asks that you simply act "as if" you had strong willpower! Simple as that. Think of how a person with strong willpower would act in that situation. Then, simply "act as if" you were that person. You'll find that you had strong willpower all along. You just didn't know it.

We find we're not slaves to our emotions. Our willpower can give us the freedom we need to act our own lives and to think, feel and behave precisely as we choose.

It's as Lincoln said, "We are as happy as we make up our minds to be." More contemporary suggestions might be: direct your feet to the sunny side of the street, put on a happy face, and let a smile be your umbrella.

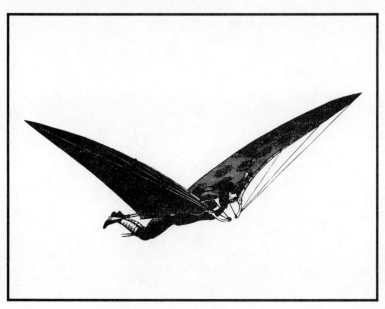

The Program

Do at least three of every one of these exercises every day for the next thirty days. In other words, three per day, thirty days, ninety exercises. Keep track of your homework in the log pages at the end of the book. By the time you've ended the month you'll be a new person. Your willpower will be stronger and more responsive.

As you practice these exercises in your daily life, you'll soon learn that they work with surprising speed to strengthen your willpower and give you the edge you need to stick to your diet. As you carry out these exercises, remember that you are applying the principle of building strength of willpower. Follow the instructions and try the exercises even though they may seem, at first, impractical to you. No matter how abstract or impractical, you will learn they can unlock your willpower and help you to achieve the goal you desire.

*By annihilating the desires,
you annihilate the mind.
Every man without passions
has within him
no principle of action,
nor motive to act.*

—Helvetius

Building Willpower by Building Intensity

The next step in building strong, effective willpower is building willpower *intensity*, the motivating force which turns you from dieting loser to winner. This dynamic force is the direct result of desire. And when fanned by the flames of imagination, strong desire enables your willpower to achieve any task you set before it.

Desire is an emotion, an eagerness or excitement of the mind directed toward the attainment of your goal and is precedent to every action of willpower. The fact that you *have* desires, that you *want* to become thin, is evidence that they are meant to become reality. "There is nothing capricious in nature," said Emerson, "and the implanting of a desire indicates that its gratification is in the constitution of the creature that feels it." In other words, you wouldn't have a desire to lose weight unless you were capable of satisfying it.

In his book *Think and Grow Rich*, author Napoleon Hill emphasized the role desire plays in building willpower. "Everything man creates and acquires," said Hill, "begins in the form of desire. That desire is taken on the first lap of its journey from the abstract to the concrete in the workshop of the imagination, where plans for its transition are created and organized."

If you are to be successful at dieting, your reasons must be forceful and compelling; your commitment must be deep and genuine. You must want to lose weight permanently. You must want this goal earnestly, actively, vigorously, constantly, and persistently. If you want to become thin in such a degree as to *demand* a response from your willpower, then your willpower simply cannot refuse.

A Price to Pay

Many dieters don't have sufficient desire to win the weight-loss battle. Yes, they covet the slimmer bodies they see in the locker room, just as they covet the better looking cars in the company parking lot. Certainly they'd like to have one just like it. But frankly, they do not desire the better body dearly enough to pay the price to get one.

Frequently in my weight-loss classes, I have met men and women who demonstrated half-hearted belief in their reasons for becoming slim. This was particularly true for those who were only slightly overweight, say 5 to 15 pounds. Often, their attitude was that they "didn't look so bad," but thought it "might" be nice to lose "a few" pounds . . . to give my program "a try."

Shallow commitment like this cannot stand up against the barriers to losing weight permanently. Research has proven this to be true. Dieters who are only slightly overweight or borderline obese have a much more difficult time achieving their "ideal" weight than their more corpulent counterparts. The reason is obvious: Greater obesity often engenders greater *desire* to become thin.

Building Desire

Desire takes its degree of strength from the apparent importance of its object. If you want your goal badly enough, your willpower is greatly enhanced. If you don't, your will-

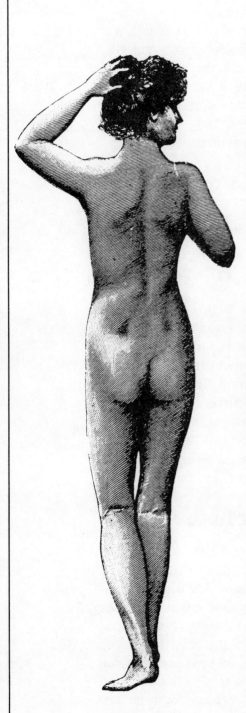

power will be as responsive as your grandmother is to acid rock.

A few dieters I've met seem to naturally possess the kind of unshakeable desire that allows them to stick to their diet without serious breakdown. These lucky souls simply refuse to accept defeat as anything more than a temporary condition, and one which urges them on to efforts even more supreme. They're the ones whose desire to succeed is so intense they can accept nothing else but victory.

A far greater number come upon their unflappable desire as the result of a cataclysmic event. I am reminded here of the many stories I have read about or have personally witnessed in which men and women have overcome great handicaps to achieve their goals. We frequently read in the newspapers and news magazines about their superhuman exploits:

A young girl crippled by a tragic car crash on the eve of her high school graduation learns to walk with the aid of new computer technology. A paraplegic teaches herself to paint like the masters holding her brush between her teeth. A young man without feet competes in the famous Ironman Triathalon in Hawaii which includes a grueling ocean swim of 2.4 miles, a hot, dusty 112-mile bicycle race, and then a heart-stopping 26.2-mile marathon.

There are quite literally millions of examples of men and women who, when cruelly dealt a handicapping blow from fate, overcome burdens so unimaginably difficult that the able-bodied shrink at their mere thought. Their desire was so forceful and compelling that they simply *refused* to be overwhelmed by temporary defeat, even predicted failure. They made up their minds that they had to achieve victory at all costs.

The Nearness of You

Most dieters, however, build the desire they need to diet successfully the old-fashioned way: They *earn it*. Through natural accretion or studied effort, they build their desire to head off the problems that plague most beginning dieters with unrelenting malevolence.

For example, the desire to achieve weight-loss goals can easily be dimmed when the goal is distant in time and space. Losing weight may often appear less important when contrasted with the great time and effort which is necessary to produce it. The nearness of the present desire—eating—dims the larger value of the slim physique, further removed.

When that happens, the pleasures of eating for today are purchased at an exorbitant price which must be paid at some future date. It's an old story: A chocolate-chip cookie held close to the eye will always seem larger than the moon.

Quantifying Your Desire

There are all kinds of reasons why dieters ought to lose weight permanently and I could easily parade at least a dozen before your captive eyes. I could talk about how losing weight will improve your health, or your appearance, mobility, sex life, and so on. But I'm going to resist that opportunity to pad this book by simply saying this: It's the reason that you believe is important that counts. And whatever reasons you choose are OK with me, just so long as they work for you.

So whether you want to hook up with a new lover, become

more pleasing and pretty to yourself, win the Miss America pageant, or become a steamily handsome *Playgirl* centerfold, it makes no difference to me. If your reasons are important to *you*, they'll sustain your willpower and help you stick to your diet.

Never mind that I'll never be able to use the nifty quote by Thomas Moffett who so wisely said, "Men dig their graves with their own teeth and die more by those instruments than the weapons of their enemies." I'll use it in some other book. Instead, let's use this valuable space helping you crystalize your reasons—whatever they may be—for going on your next (and last) diet.

List Your Reasons

Right now, scare up a piece of paper and a Bic that works and make your own personal list of reasons why you want to stick to your diet and stay thin forever. When you have at least ten, write them down in a notebook. Keep them handy. You'll have two uses for that list. Right now, you'll need it to begin doing the important imagination exercises. Later on you'll use the list in one of your exercises which builds persistence.

HOW YOUR WILLPOWER
BUILDS WILLPOWER

Your willpower uses the laws of imagination to help achieve success, universal principles that have worked for all men and women through the ages:

Law 1.

The mental images and ideas you hold in your mind tend to produce the *physical* reality and the activities to which the images correspond.

Since laws of nature always come in pairs, here is its partner:

Law 2.

A human being always acts in accordance with the mental images and ideas s/he holds and accepts, whether they are true or false, real or imagined, and regardless of their source.

"The imagination," according to Napoleon Hill, "is literally the workshop wherein are fashioned all plans created by man. The impulse, the desire, is given shape, form and action through the aid of the imagination faculty of the mind."

What Hill is saying is that, before we may really "do" anything, we must first have an image of that act already alive in our imagination. And, according to universal Law #1, once the image or idea of the thing has been created, then willpower will see to it that the *physical* counterpart to the thing is created. You'll enable your willpower to create its counterpart in reality, a slim, new, youthful body.

We see evidence everywhere that this is true. Whenever we have an idea which we think about constantly, our minds cannot help churning out ideas and actions to turn that idea into reality. A better job. A more workable relationship with your spouse or children. A better way of doing things. If we can *imagine* the answer to our problem, we can *create* the answer.

The second principle is even more important than the first. This law states, in effect, that a person always acts, feels and performs in accordance with the images in his or her mind, regardless of where they come from. When you think and believe in yourself as a "winner," for example, thoughts and ideas that support your belief are filtered from the ideas and images about you. Those which are appropriate to your mindset are allowed entrance. Ideas that do not match your mindset are discarded.

Moreover, the law says, the mind *never* acts in a vacuum. It will process *any* thoughts and ideas it receives from wherever it gets them. The subconscious mind makes no distinction whatsoever between constructive and destructive thought images. Nor does it judge whether the material it receives is true or false, real or imagined.

But the more important point is this: The subconscious will do this with any information it gets, even images which you purposefully plant in your subconscious.

Keep repeating to your son that he is stupid and worthless and, before long, he'll reproduce that image in reality. In other words, he'll start behaving as if he were stupid and worthless. He'll start selecting and accepting from his world those images and ideas that support his worthlessness.

On the other hand, tell a student he is exceptionally bright, and although he may have only average intelligence, he'll begin to perform according to the new image of himself which he perceives. He'll begin to perform better than average.

Again, remember it makes no difference whether the image is true or false. If you *perceive* it to be true, it carries full weight.

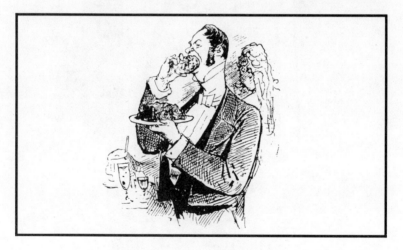

Food for Thought

Feed your mind thoughts about brownies, ice cream, and dieting failure, and "whatsoever a man soweth, that shall he also reap." You'll soon be bingeing on ice cream and brownies.

Feed it thoughts about slimness, approval, and a happier life, and your mind will find harmonizing thoughts and ideas

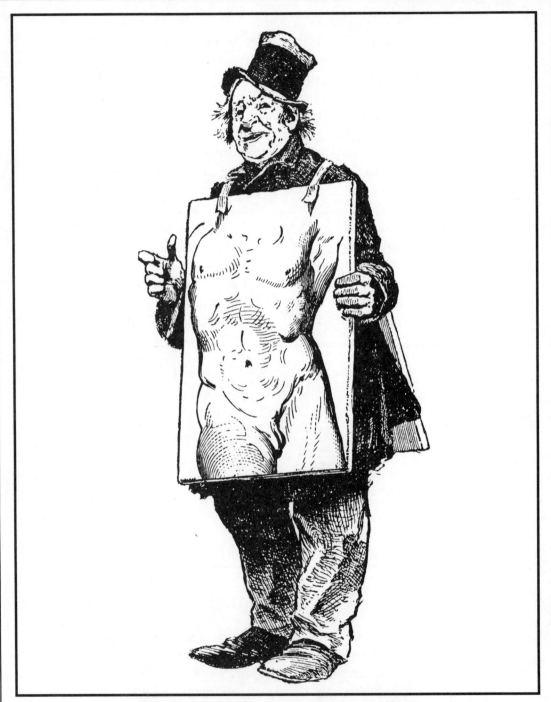

When losing weight, imagination is everything.

from the world around it to turn these thoughts into the real thing: a permanently thinner you.

Think of yourself as a dieting loser, and you'll become a dieting loser. But think of yourself as a winner and the winner's circle will soon be yours!

Why Not *Imagine* Yourself as Thin and Beautiful?

Realizing that your actions, feelings, and behavior are the result of the images and beliefs you provide your mind, you have the perfect tool you need to build your willpower and win the weight-loss battle.

By evoking mental pictures of yourself as successfully dieting and maintaining a slimmer figure, you'll provide yourself with the images your willpower needs to turn these images into a reality.

EXERCISE 1.
SHARPENING YOUR IMAGINATION

Every day for the next thirty days, I want you to do just that. Set aside a time each day when you can relax, uninterrupted. A time when you can let your imagination run free and wild.

You might choose to do this exercise in the morning, before you arise from bed, or perhaps at the end of the day before you go to sleep. Any comfortable spot will do: a bed, a couch, an easy chair, even at your desk. Allow yourself to become as relaxed as possible. Close your eyes and let your thoughts drift inward.

Your First Week
During the first seven days of this exercise, picture as vividly as you can how developing a strong and powerful will

can make your life more rewarding, more satisfying.

Think of how you will behave when you have a strong and powerful will. Think of your achievements. Make these pictures as detailed as possible. Are you confident and self-assured? Are you achieving success in the areas of your life where it matters?

See yourself acting confidently and deliberately in those situations which previously have brought you chaos and despair. See yourself behaving with assuredness, poise, and above all, *determination* where you may have previously wilted with trepidation.

Hold these pictures in your mind as long as you can. Turn them over again and again. Look for new detail, added dimension, colorful nuance, and particularly, rich emotions.

When mixed with emotions your mental pictures literally come alive in your imagination. I'm thinking about emotions such as love, happiness, joy, etc. When you drench your images with these emotions they are twice as valuable as willpower-building devices. How do you *feel* when you're "under control"? Confident? Self-assured? Happy? What emotions do you experience when you use a powerful will?

Since this technique is new to most of you, it will take time and practice to gain its most important results. Your powers of imagination may have grown weak from disuse. But your imagination, just like your willpower, can become more alert through use, just as any muscle or organ of the body becomes stronger through use.

Week Two

During the second seven days of this exercise, follow the instructions above, but this time, project images about achieving your dieting goals and think how this important success will improve your life. Think about how you'll look when you're thinner, for example. Your new, shapelier figure. Your new confidence and poise.

What clothes are you wearing? In what new activities are

you participating? What is your attitude? Are you confident and self-assured? Pay attention to every detail of sight, sound, and sense.

Be particularly careful to search for visions which reflect your reasons for dieting and be sure to add the special leavening agent of *emotion*. Think not only in terms of being thin, but "happily" and "joyously" thin. Or thin and "sexy." You know what I mean.

Imagine each benefit in its smallest detail so that you become thoroughly familiar with every aspect of the idea. By so doing, you will set for yourself a pattern, or create a mold, after which your dieting life will shape itself. You will create well-beaten mental paths, "habits" as it were, along which your willpower can travel in its search for shapely expression. Repeat the same visual pictures, the same "movie" again and again, and a new dieting life will take shape before your very eyes.

There is no need at this point for you to think about how you're going to become thin. Believe me, when you repeatedly imagine yourself successfully thin, the "how" will *automatically* take care of itself.

Third and Fourth Weeks

In the third and fourth week, these imagination exercises grow longer, first to twenty minutes and then thirty minutes. Think about how your strong and powerful willpower can produce the visions of loveliness. See yourself moving about with poise and grace. How your willpower can routinely say "no" to caloric temptations and how much better you'll look because you can now do this successfully.

It Works!

Successful dieters have profited from this technique over and over again. A thirty-year-old advertising agency secretary told me her story:

"I'm not quite sure why it works, but it worked wonders for me. I had been overweight since junior high school and every time I tried to diet, it seemed I would get depressed at some point about my lack of progress and then I'd quit.

"When I finally made up my mind to get rid of my unwanted weight, I tried the imagination technique. I was already familiar with it because I had recently read about it in a book. Although I was skeptical I tried it. And just like they said, controlling myself became easier. I really began to believe in myself and my ability to get thin. Each time I did the exercise I thought of new ways to make my diet work better. I have no idea why it works. It just works."

The book that Meg referred to was the best-selling *Psycho-Cybernetics* by Maxwell Maltz. In Maltz's book, he recounts the miracles that many men and women have achieved by building willpower through imagination. His work cites how a salesman increased his sales 400 percent by simply *imagining* he was successful; how a world-famous chess player and a professional golfer "practiced" winning plays in their imagination; how a renowned concert pianist practiced the piano "in his head."

Napoleon Hill has written of many more such examples. Hill, Atkinson, Assagioli, and many other famous students of willpower before them, recognized the vital role that imagination plays in increasing desire and building willpower, whether "success" is defined as losing weight forever or making a million dollars.

This daily exercise will fan the flames of desire, sending new determination and resoluteness to your willpower. These visions, rich with desire-supporting emotions, also will become new memories, new "tapes" if you will, that your willpower can play when your diet needs a temporary boost. Before long, you'll see yourself spontaneously acting with new confidence and poise. You'll find that you can diet effortlessly, successfully.

Imagination Brings Dieting Success

H. Jon Geis of New York City's Institute for Rational Living is one of hundreds of dieting specialists who agrees that dieters become more successful in their weight-loss efforts if they bring to their mind's eye a vivid picture of their dieting success. Geis advises you to keep these ideas and images of dieting success in your mind at all times, and think of them frequently during the day. Often, he says, you will find a thought or picture flashing through your mind just when you need the extra spark of willpower.

EXERCISE 2. WORDS OF POWER

Another exercise which is quite successful in developing your desire is called "words of power." The secret here is to think of the *words* which produce vivid images of dieting and willpower success. Only you can provide the words, since only you know which words have the power to evoke strong, positive mental images of your success.

One word which works especially well for me is "winner." I'm not exactly sure why but this word produces a rich variety of vivid mental images every time I use it. But then again, who doesn't like to be told he or she is a winner?

Another word I like is simply "success." Perhaps in your mind these two words mean the same thing but to me they elicit entirely different images.

To bring these words alive in your imagination, get a sheet of lined paper and write your "word of power" as many times as you can. My guess is you'll write the word anywhere from two hundred to four hundred times.

As you begin what appears to be a genuinely tedious task, an interesting thing happens. Your mind will start drifting from the mechanical labor of writing the word and you'll unconsciously start forming images of what your word of power means to you.

You'll start daydreaming about how much more sexy and attractive you'll look when you're thin. About the clothes you'll wear. About the places you'll go. About the people you'll meet and how they'll feel about you. Think about these images and keep writing. They'll keep coming just as long as you keep writing.

It's a fabulous exercise. Try it and you'll see! You can also use your words of power as you think about dieting during the day. Just thinking about your power words can begin the flow of desire-building images.

SELECTING YOUR "POWER" WORDS

Right now make up a list of a half-dozen "power" words for your dieting vocabulary. Maybe "skinny" or "trim" or "attractive" are the words that light up your desire. Maybe the words you select will have nothing to do with dieting. So be it.

My Personal Words of Power

1. _____

2. _____

3. _____

4. _____

5. _____

6. _____

7. _____

8. _____

9. _____

10. _____

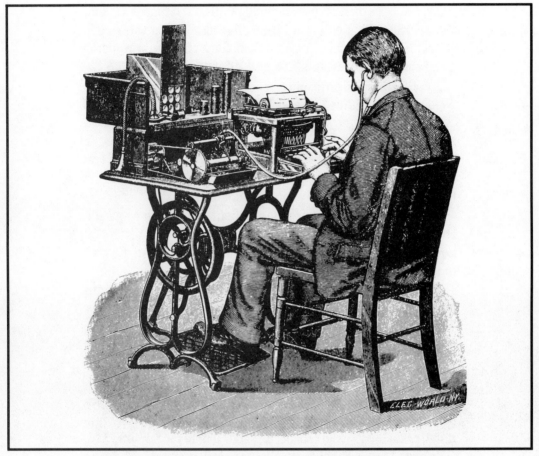

An easy way to keep track of your dieting Words of Power.

EXERCISE 3.
BOOKS THAT BUILD DESIRE

Your desire of will can also be developed by learning of the willpower-building activities of others. Here are some of the books I'd recommend as being useful in your attempt to build a strong, enthusiastic will.

Psycho-Cybernetics, by Maxwell Maltz. I referred to this book earlier. This perennial bestseller has helped thousands of people just like you improve their lives through a remarkable program of exercises to build self-image.

Another book I'd recommend as a terrific stem-winder is *The Power of Positive Thinking* by Norman Vincent Peale. This easy-to-read volume will contribute handsomely to your dieting success by teaching how to build desire, as I do in this book. We both teach that success is in *your* hands. And if you make up your mind that your will be done, there's nothing on this Earth that can stop you. It *will* be yours.

Still another book which is excellent reading is Napoleon Hill's *Think and Grow Rich*. This upbeat work will teach you how to take a new look at yourself and give you a realistic way to achieve your goals whatever they may be.

And you can immeasurably speed the progress of strengthening your willpower by reading *How to Get Control of Your Time and Your Life* by Arthur Lakein. Lakein's practical guide shows you how to choose, prioritize and plan short- and long-term goals, and organize your life. All of these are important steps in the willpower building process.

You might also choose any one of a number of good biographies about outstanding men and women. Contemporary illuminati such as Lee Iacocca, Ted Turner, Sandra Day O'Connor, etc., provide excellent moral support. There is something about reading about the success of others that strengthens your will to achieve. Reading, and the images it creates, awakens the vast inner energy within you which has long been dormant just waiting for such a revival.

I'm sure you may have other favorites. Why not go to your library today and choose a couple of these books for your nightly reading project for the next thirty days? Books like these are tremendously effective in building willpower. And I urge you to start reading today.

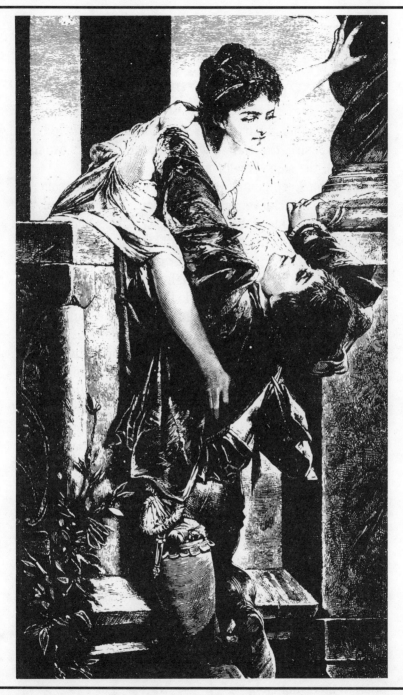

When you reach your dieting goal, all sorts of wonderful things can happen.

EXERCISE 4. KEEPING COMPANY
WITH THE WINNERS

Just as *reading* about the success of others can help build willpower desire, *associating* with successful others can also accomplish the same beneficial purpose.

When you keep company with winning dieters, some of their desire to achieve rubs off on you. That's one of the reasons why dieting clubs like Weight Watchers and Overeaters Anonymous claim to have higher rates of permanent weight-loss for their members over dieters who try to go it alone. And let's face it, losing weight is a lonely business. All too often the dieter gets little or no help from his or her family and friends. I realize these people want to help, but frankly, they really don't know *how* to support your diet.

To strengthen your willpower, seek out supportive dieting friends who share your desire to become thin. Wherever you live there are dieting clubs and organizations that serve this important purpose. The winners in these groups are successful models for your continued dieting. It is very reassuring to know that others have made huge sacrifices to stay on their diets; that their struggles are your struggles; that none of you is alone. When you see that sticking to a diet is both possible and rewarding, you'll begin to see, feel and *believe* that you can do it too!

A word of caution, however. Joining a diet club is no guarantee you'll *stay* in one. Dieting club members suffer from the same lack of willpower that plagues dieters as a whole. In fact, the *majority* of dieters drop out of these clubs at rates comparable to those who fail to stick to their diets. It's been estimated that 80 percent of those who join dieting clubs dropout in the first six months. It's the same story over again. They lack a well-trained willpower to stick to their diet or stick to their diet club.

Staying in a diet club, though, works wonders—if you have

a willpower to do it. Dr. Robert M. Johnson, chairman of the board of the American Society of Bariatric Physicians (doctors who specialize in obesity) agrees, saying persistence here pays off.

"If you beat the odds," says Johnson, "the chances are that whatever group you stick with will help you lose weight." And he adds a useful postscript: "You're more likely to stay in the group where you feel most comfortable."

Practice Makes Perfect

As you practice these exercises each day, you'll be amazed at how quickly they'll incite your desire to the levels which successful dieting requires. These are exercises which you can perform at any time, and for any goal. And they'll continue to work just as long as you continue to use them.

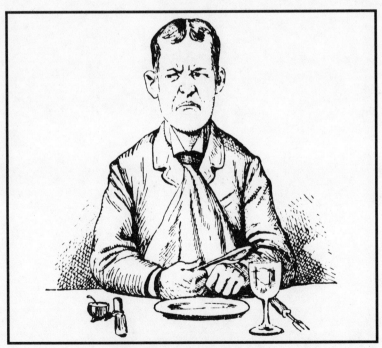

Dieting alone is never fun.

> *When a man knows*
> *he is to be hanged*
> *in a fortnight,*
> *it concentrates his mind*
> *wonderfully.*
>
> —Samuel Johnson

Building Willpower through Better Concentration

It often begins so innocently. The dieter is hungry, and this hunger automatically triggers those "little sentences" to start flowing through your mind. Words and phrases like "cookies," or "brownies" and that ever-popular, "pie à la mode."

Pretty soon we begin arguing with ourselves about whether to actually start eating cookies, brownies, or ice cream. And then your strength of will is put to the acid test: "Should I or shouldn't I?" And you remember who usually wins that battle.

If only you could find a way to imprison these maverick little thoughts when they start, maybe they wouldn't grow into the full-blown threat that they do. If only you could think about only what you truly want to think about.

Well, there is a way.

Concentration is a willpower quality which works to keep your mind's attention firmly fixed upon the object of your willpower: your goal.

Concentration refers to your willpower's ability to *retain* and display images and ideas which help achieve your willpower goal and the mind's ability to *remove* or inhibit the display of images and ideas which threaten your willpower goal.

Concentration is needed in all kinds of training, from athletics to musicianship. And it's particularly important to dieters. In fact, this power might be second in importance only to strength in helping you to achieve your weight-loss goals. Without it, self-control is impossible. And as Pythagoras said, "No man is free who cannot command himself."

Concentration Can Save Your Next Diet

The reason this quality is important is obvious: The impulse to eat is mainly triggered by a host of conditioned thoughts which, when given even temporary freedom, spread like oil on water throughout your mind.

Dieters who lack such control over marauding thoughts are given to daydreaming about food and eating. As these fantasies flit about the caverns of their mind, however, they can grow and become stronger, more forceful. And when they do, you'll find yourself in the midst of self-argument. "Should I, or shouldn't I?" But by then, your diet is usually doomed.

Now, if you pit the strength of your will *directly* against the wayward thought, you are likely to fail. But if you use a skillful, less forcible method by deliberately creating a different center of attention, you can easily liberate your captive attention and escape from the situation unscathed.

And isn't that the biggest problem when you give up anything? It's not bad enough you had to "do without" the cigarettes, coffee, alcohol, or high-calorie food you're trying to give up, you're also bombarded with thoughts and visions of the forbidden fruits.

The Winning Strategy

A strong power of concentration can *withdraw* the mind's eye from objects and ideas which interfere with its chosen course. The process is called "inhibition," and it's not to be confused with what you lose at the office Christmas party after four martinis.

When you're fully occupied with matters unrelated to cheating, bingeing, "giving in," etc., you block out thoughts of food and eating.

Thus, the effective strategy is this: When you're confronted by an impulse to cheat on your diet, willpower diminishes the impulse by turning your attention and involvement to other things. By consciously interrupting your focus of attention and resisting the lure of daydreaming about food, you can temporarily get over a difficult situation. The lure of cheating is thereby knocked out before it gets down to the stage where bareknuckled fighting by willpower strength gets involved. And as important as strength is, I think you'll agree that it's better to avoid these kinds of fights whenever possible. Will-power concentration can help build this kind of dieting control.

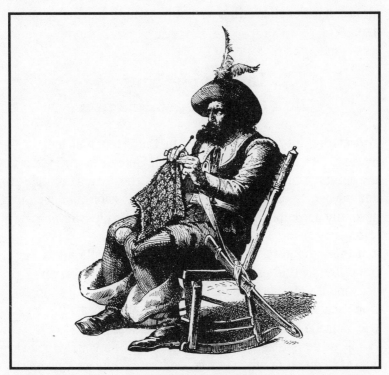

Keeping busy keeps thoughts of cheating out of your mind.

One of the easiest ways to control your mind is keep busy. Keep your mind off the culinary themes which can destroy your dieting resolve. Obviously, if your mind is occupied on thoughts unrelated to food, it can't also be thinking about eating. Or to put it another way, a busy person never knows how much he or she weighs.

The ability to focus our thoughts on a single subject or idea can be easily improved by doing just that: by paying strict attention to the idea. But that's not always easy to do. Let's face it, this is the real world we live in, not "Life With Father." Divorces, accidents, death, and myriad woes await our every step to grieve us.

Equally disruptive to the lives of dieters are happy occasions. Good fortune can easily be construed as cause for celebration and cheating on your dieting plans, "just for now." Thus, whether the events of life bless or grieve us, the dieter's mind can rationalize either as justification to scuttle his or her diet.

Improving Your
Powers of Concentration

Actually, all of the exercises in this book will help willpower in its quest for concentration. Since concentration is the ability to bring to our mind exactly those thoughts, ideas, and psychological forces which we desire, each time we purposefully accomplish such an attempt our willpower becomes stronger.

Take the ability to effectively imagine, for instance. Each time you do this exercise you are purposefully bringing to your mind's eye thoughts and visions of your dieting success. And each time you do that, your ability to concentrate in this way is made more powerful, more effective.

The same is true when you concentrate on your willpower goal statement, or when you concentrate while writing one of your Words of Power. And the better you can concentrate, the more you can control the tempting thoughts and ideas that often crowd your mind.

But there are other exercises that build concentration as well. Among them are goal setting, purposefully changing your focus of attention, and focusing on the uninteresting. First, a word about setting goals.

Building Concentration through Goal-Setting

Goals are the mental roadmaps which your willpower uses to attain its desired ends, the conduits that funnel all of your physical and mental energies toward a single, important purpose.

A wealth of professional research has proven that goal setting helps improve your ability to concentrate and, therefore, your ability to stick to your diet. Writing in the *Canadian Journal of Behavioral Science*, for example, researchers Pierre Baron and Robert G. Watters revealed that dieters who set goals lose much more weight than those who do not.

Their findings confirm scores of earlier studies including those by Robert L. Litrownik of the University of Illinois, H. Jon Geis of the Institute for Rational Living, New York City, and others. All verify that the ability to stick to your diet and achieve weight-loss success is aided considerably by proper goal-setting.

How Goal-Setting Builds Willpower

Goal setting builds willpower because it works in precisely the same way as your imagination exercises work: Both rely on the mind's ability to turn thoughts into *things*, ideas into successful reality.

Goal-setting the "Weight Loss through Willpower" way keeps your diet at the forefront of your daily dietary thinking. The result is that you're constantly reminded in a positive, forceful way that dieting is your top priority, a daily routine to which you devote unswerving allegiance.

Your goal becomes your mental companion as you steadily chip away at those unwanted pounds. It measures your successes, complements your achievements, redirects your efforts from past mistakes and false starts.

EXERCISE 1.
SETTING PERFECT GOALS

Five Easy Steps for Perfect Goal-Setting

There are five easy rules for setting effective goals. Anybody can do it. You need only take a half-hour or so, do a bit of soul-searching and pencil work, and *voilà*, 'tis *fait accompli*.

Step One

Fix in your mind the *exact* goal you wish to reach. Be as definite as possible, but beware: Do not get caught in the trap of setting a goal for one thing when you really want another.

Many overweight people diet because they want to "get thin" but their real goal is not to get thin, it's to stay thin. That's like climbing Mt. Everest when your goal was really to build a six-room condo up there. Since the strategies involved in "losing weight" and "staying thin permanently" are quite different, you can understand why the precious few who reach their ideal weight will often complain later that the weight came back.

So get it right the first time. If you want to lose fifteen pounds, say so. If you want to lose fifty pounds and remain at 110 for the rest of your life—admit it and be proud. If you want to lose twenty pounds and eat nutritionally better meals, make that decision. But above all, *be definite*. Tell your willpower exactly what you want, and your willpower will find a way to make it happen.

Step Two

Determine exactly *how* you are going to achieve this goal. This step of goal-setting calls for some planning on your part since you've got to know the wherefores of choosing a particular diet, what the likely results will be, and what action you'll take if this diet runs into a snag.

Unfortunately, most dieters are impulsive to a fault. They slip into new diets more frequently than Joan Collins takes on new lovers. And, perhaps, with about as much thought.

Planning is that principle through which you organize a definite plan to achieve your goal; a plan which forms the heart of your weight-loss program and which includes *alternative* procedures in case your diet runs aground.

The problem is that most dieters let other people think and plan for them. They turn over their problems in hopes that someone else might solve them. They accept the opinions and decisions of others and imagine that they themselves are thinking. They only *think* that they think. Emerson noted this when he said, "Our chief want in life is somebody who will make us do what we can."

So a word of preachy caution: Don't shirk your dieting responsibility. Make it your problem. Sure, you could start with the broad outlines of one of the popular "bookstore diets." But then why not customize it and make it your own? Remember you'll never be a dieting winner if you think somebody else is responsible for making you get thin.

Step Three

Select a *timetable* for the attainment of your goal. This will take some calculations on your part, predicting the rate of pounds lost through caloric restriction and increased physical activity.

Setting a timetable is important. It is difficult to make firm connections between the fading past and unseen future if you don't have a timetable to plot your course. To make this association more explicit, keep a logbook of your dieting progress. Although these dieting diaries are sometimes viewed as tedious pencil-pushing, they're valuable in charting your progress, reviving spirits that flag, and motivation that founders. Besides, they're always a rush to read in later months or years.

But with or without a daily weight record, your frequent weigh-ins will keep you aware of your progress. Based upon the degree of your intermediate successes, you can reward yourself or deliver consequences to yourself and adopt the self-correcting behavior you'll need to achieve your goal on schedule.

Step Four

Make a fresh commitment as to what you'll do to prevent a relapse in your weight-loss program. To accomplish this step you'll need to deliberate and make contracts with yourself.

Much of what you have done in your dieting past has been correct. You need only repeat your past dieting successes to bring you closer to victory next time.

But what about those areas in which you've had problems? Do you, for example, have problems sticking to your diet during holiday entertaining? Are you particularly vulnerable

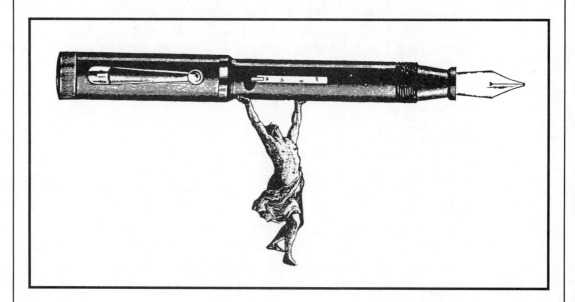

to dieting failure when you eat in a restaurant? Have you stumbled and fallen on your road to a slimmer you as the result of a temporary personal problem, depression, anxiety, anger, etc.?

Whatever the problem, you've got to *preplan* its solution, in case it arises in your dieting life again. What will you do differently next time? Make a note of that action and include it in your goal statement.

Step Five

The fifth and final step is to reduce your four goal statements into *writing*. Read this written goal statement aloud to yourself three or more times daily and, for certain, once in the morning when you first wake up; again just before you go to bed at night. As you read your goal, see and feel and *believe* you have already reached your weight-loss goal.

Here's what your goal statement might look like:

> *"I am going to lose twenty-five pounds (you're specific) by April 15 by undertaking the Pritikin Diet and by jogging thirty minutes a day at least four days a week. If I fail to jog four days a week or cheat on my diet by more than one hundred calories, I will do an added hour of exercise."*

Read this statement out loud to yourself at least three times a day. Memorize it. This is one of the most important psychological steps of effective willing that you can undertake.

The Magic of Auto-Suggestion

What you are practicing in Step Five is the principle of auto-suggestion: your direct link of communication with your subconscious.

In our chapter on building willpower intensity, I repeatedly noted the role of imagination in building your desire to stick to your diet, lose weight, and become beautifully thin. This plan was promulgated under the laws of nature that you can feed your subconscious any and all images which you like, and your subconscious will turn these thoughts and images into their corporeal counterparts.

Auto-suggestion works in the same way. Your subconscious mind is normally not accessible to any sort of direct control from the conscious mind. However, since you do have absolute control over your conscious mind, you can repeatedly send positive thoughts and ideas to your subconscious. And in turn, the subconscious begins its mysterious process of turning those thoughts into their real life counterparts.

Each time you read your goal statement, you are sending orders to your subconscious, orders which it *must* eventually obey. And remember that your subconscious mind reacts best to these orders when they are drenched in desire-supporting emotions and any other imagery from the five senses you can provide.

EXERCISE 2. CHANGING YOUR FOCUS OF ATTENTION

Take any feeling or emotion that you are experiencing at this moment, and turn your attention away from it and on to something else. Use your willpower to concentrate on the other thought and pay no attention whatsoever to the unwanted one.

You'll probably find your attention is a little rebellious at first. It wants to fly back to the unwanted thought. But keep your willpower fixed firmly upon the task.

Hold your attention upon the other thing. Examine all facets and nuances of the thought. Before long, an amazing thing will begin to happen: Your attention will grow increasingly interested in the new thought and less and less interested in the old one. In a short time the other thought or feeling will have disappeared.

The popular way of describing this process would be: "Keep your mind off it." And with a little practice, you can keep your mind on or off anything you desire. Remember, willpower is the master of the mental states. And attention is the key to the process.

EXERCISE 3. FOCUSING ATTENTION ON THE UNINTERESTING

Anyone can devote attention to an interesting thing. But it takes a highly trained willpower to place and hold attention upon an uninteresting one.

In our final exercise, rather than fastening attention on just any thought other than the one currently in your mind, this exercise specifically requires focusing attention on a particularly uninteresting idea.

Few people can deliberately fasten their attention upon some dry subject, and then hold it there with willpower. And yet such a quality is a frequent requisite for the man or woman who would succeed with a diet.

Find some dry idea and fasten your attention upon the idea for increasingly longer periods of time. First just two or three minutes. Then growing to five, ten, and fifteen.

As you do this exercise you'll notice that it becomes easier and easier to do. Our willpower continually disciplines us until such tasks become easy to do.

What Concentration Exercises Do for You

By performing these exercises once or twice daily for thirty days, you will find that your powers of concentration are dramatically improved. You'll find that you can switch and move your attention from subject to subject at will. And thus when you get into those tight corners where an internal war is raging in your mind over "should I or shouldn't I," you'll be able to brush aside that line of thinking, recover your poise, and continue your diet.

*And you shall
know the truth,
And the truth
shall set you free.*

—John 8:32

Building Willpower Confidence

It is no secret that belief in your ability to succeed can significantly contribute to your power to succeed. There is no doubt whatsoever that confidence may even be one of the most important attributes of willpower.

If you took the quiz in Chapter 3 and found yourself undecided as to whether or not you could win the weight-loss battle once and for all, this chapter is for you.

It is through faith that all things are made possible including losing weight forever. Keyserling has said, "Only that inward affirmation which is called faith creates the decision which 'makes real' the self in phenomenal existence." Or as recorded in St. Mark, "All things are possible to him that believeth."

But what is confidence? In its simplest form, it is belief that is not based upon evidence or proof.

We reach our convictions in one of two ways. First, we may reach a conviction through mental intelligence. That is, we become convinced of the truth or falsity of a proposition because we mentally deduce the principles upon which it is founded.

I am convinced, for example, that the sun will rise tomorrow morning even though I may not actually see it. I understand the general principles of science and celestial bodies in space thanks to a long, and often boring, class in college astronomy.

On the other hand, I also know I can become a doctor or lawyer, learn to speak fluent French or Spanish, or become a world-class marathon runner. I am convinced of these things not because I have done them, and not because I have studied and deduced the priniciples of language development or the mechanics of the running body.

I know I can do them because I intuit their possibility. That is, I recognize that, although I have never done these things, they are in harmony with what I perceive as my true nature. In short, I have *faith* that I can accomplish these things.

I know enough about my personal abilities and the requirements of achieving these goals to "know" that I can accomplish them.

These two kinds of convictions—intellectual and intuitive faith—are within us in varying degrees and in varying proportions all the time. It is through a combination of intellectual conviction and intuition that we reach what might be called a *certainty*.

Certainty is a state in which the dieter believes in his or her ability to lose weight because he or she knows and understands the principles upon which dieting and metabolism are founded; and a faith which comes from knowing that losing weight and staying thin harmonize with the dieter's understanding of his or her past performances. Past performance, together with current evidence, leads to confidence in the outcome of things. This dual state of certainty is what you're looking for.

The mental reasoning that men and women can lose weight and achieve permanent weight loss is readily apparent. But you may have a hard time accepting, through faith, the proposition that *you* can lose weight permanently. After all, you have tried to stay on your diet again and again. Each time you have failed. What reason convinced you that you'll win this time?

Research Says You Can

Successful dieters often tell me that when they finally surrendered to their diet and decided to lose weight permanently, they experienced a corresponding burst of faith in their ability to do so. Suddenly, where they had been merely passengers on their ship of fate, they were the captains. And nothing would stand in their way of success.

Considerable research has confirmed their experiences and the crucial role of confidence in dieting success. Typical of such research is that of Kevin J. Hartigan and researchers at the Illinois Institute of Technology. These scientists documented the relationship between *belief* in one's ability to lose weight and the actual weight loss the dieters achieved.

The results were dramatic. Dieting confidence, they found, is one of the most important predictors of your ability to lose weight. In fact in some individuals, it could be *the* most important factor. *Così è se vi pare.* Right you are if you think you are.

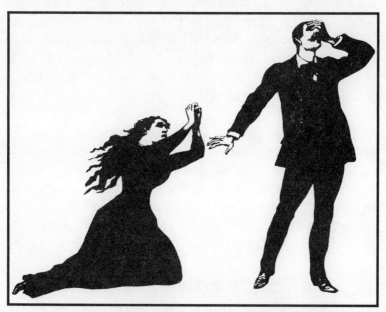

"I promise. If you let me watch Wheel of Fortune, I'll stop eating Ding-Dongs."

On the other hand, notice what happens when a woman says to herself, "I have failed three times to stick to my diet," and what happens when a woman says, "I am a failure."

No One Is Doomed to Quit a Diet

There are millions of dieters who believe they are forever doomed to remain fat. They have tried and failed to stay on a diet so many times that their self-confidence has plummeted so low you'd need a divining rod to find it. Each successive attempt and failure to stick it out is seen as further evidence that this is true. Then it becomes a vicious circle: low self-worth produces dieting failures, and each new dieting failure produces added self-reproachment which makes staying on the next diet all the harder.

This is auto-suggestion in reverse. As I pointed out in the chapters on building strength and desire, negative thinking is a self-fulfilling prophecy. We fail because we think we'll fail.

Remember that confidence is a state of mind. What a person thinks of himself will determine, even dictate, his fate. "Determine to be something in this world," said Hawes, "and you will be something. Aim at excellence, and excellence will be attained. This is the great secret of effort and eminence. 'I cannot do it' never accomplished anything. 'I will try' has wrought wonders."

Writer Norman Vincent Peale agreed when he wrote, "If you expect failure, you will get failure. If you expect to succeed, I am sure you will succeed."

Develop, therefore, a strong faith and belief in your ability to lose weight permanently *all by yourself*. You have only to plant those fertile seeds of belief in your subconscious. Once planted they will bloom profusely into a strong, durable faith.

It's What's Inside That Counts

It's well known that we are who we are because of the thoughts and feelings which dominate our minds. Fill your mind with negative thoughts and feelings, and that's what you'll get—failure at every turn. Fill your mind with thoughts of success, and your mind will *automatically* seek to duplicate that success with its counterpart, a slimmer, more beautiful you.

Cast those negative thoughts from your mind, once and for all. Replace them with positive thoughts and feelings. We believe whatever we repeat to ourselves, whether true or false. In time, you will come to believe *any* thought you place in your mind. Just keep repeating it and your subconscious will pick up the theme, and soon all manner of harmonizing thoughts will fill your mind.

Through Faith She Reached Her Goal

As an example of this I relate the case of Kay, a forty-four-year-old post office employee who had been fat since adulthood and had repeatedly tried to lose seventy-five pounds.

She was frustrated and miserable. She felt little hope that she could ever stay on a diet and reach her weight-loss goal. But she was a person driven.

One day she was taking a summer's walk around a neighborhood lake and got on the receiving end of some merciless taunts from some kids riding their bicycles. The insults were nothing she hadn't heard before. But this time she heard them one time too often. She was mad. And she cried. She was incensed. And she vowed with the tears flowing from her eyes that she *was* going to lose weight; this time, once and for all. "I'll show those little #&*%#."

Instantly, she intuitively knew she was going to reach her weight-loss goal. Her decision was so genuine, so emotional and sincere, she just knew that she could now lose the weight she so desperately wanted to shed. No, she didn't know exactly *how*. But she knew she could. She knew she *would*.

Almost immediately, her new mindset began to *automatically* seek new harmonizing thoughts. Not the "old tapes" playing the negative tunes of yesterday. She eagerly began to

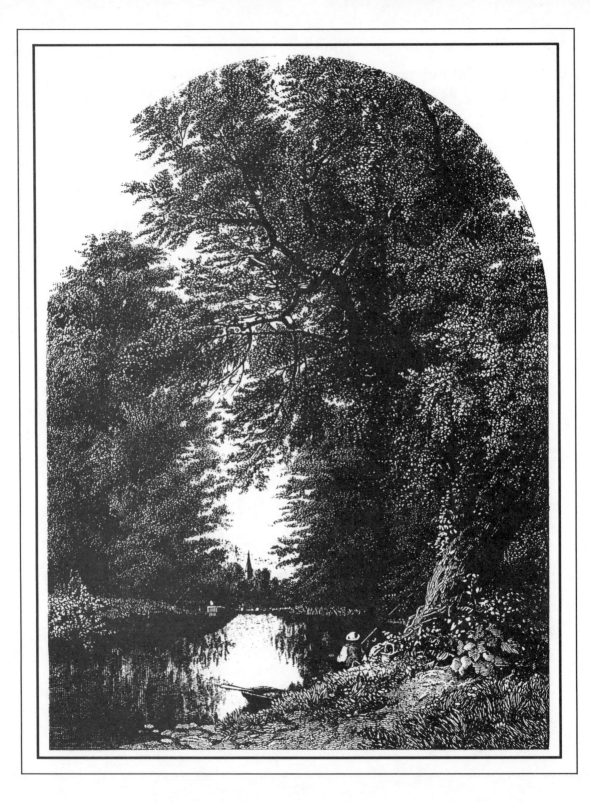

think of ways to get herself to stay on a diet and lose the weight she so deeply wanted to leave behind.

The key word here is "automatically."

How to Build Faith

Somewhere within you right now is the same sleeping giant of faith, ready to be awakened and lead your way to weight-loss success. And the way to coax the giant into action is within your mind.

You can start by ridding your mind of all negative thoughts about your past dieting failures. Resolve now to forget about past failures. You are starting over fresh, right now. The past is past and the future is yet to be. A new day is dawning that has never been used before. It's a new opportunity to start out fresh with vigor and renewed faith.

Each day is made special
By what we can give it
By how we accept it
Then how we live it.

THE FIVE STEPS OF BUILDING FAITH THROUGH THE MIRACLE OF SELF-SUGGESTION

You can begin the process of building faith with the miracle of self-suggestion. There are a number of excellent exercises which can help you do this.

1. Imagination
2. Repetition of goal statement
3. Repetitions with variations

4. Words of power

5. Act as if

Practice these principles and you'll learn to believe in yourself and your ability to achieve your goal.

1. Imagination

You have already read about the wonders that your imagination can do in creating the mental atmosphere for your continuing success. Nowhere is your imagination more important than in building faith.

Refer again to the exercises on how to use imagination to build willpower in Chapter 6. Practice these exercises daily until you are convinced you can and *will* lose your unwanted weight forever.

2. Repetition of Goal

Another way to build faith is by setting effective goals. Do you remember how that's done? Here's a refresher course.

1. State exactly how many pounds you wish to lose.

2. Determine how you're going to lose it.

3. Select a timetable for its achievement.

4. Make a commitment to prevent relapse.

5. Reduce your goal to writing and read it aloud three times a day.

Each time you perform this exercise, you're sending positive messages to your subconscious that you *will* become thin again. Repeat this goal statement to yourself as many times as you can. The more times you repeat it, the faster it will work its magic on your subconscious where plans for your dieting success are built.

The principle at work here is auto-suggestion, which we discussed at length in Chapter 7. And it's the same theory that is used by advertisers who repeat the same message to their audiences again and again to good effect. When TV viewers or radio listeners get to the store, the message which has been repeated the most often is the product they'll remember, and the one they might be more likely to buy.

Your Subconscious as Consumer

The message you're asking your subconscious to "buy" is this: "I *can* and I *will* lose this unwanted weight forever." Repeated enough times, your subconscious will accept this statement as true, and seek to duplicate its counterpart in reality.

3. Repetitions with Variations

Using the same principle, you may wish to create a series of messages to send to your subconscious. Each can be different. This will help you avoid the possibility of your message becoming monotonous and your delivery routine and hopelessly mechanical.

Here are some examples:

1. "I can and I will lose this unwanted weight forever."

2. "I know I have the ability to lose this weight permanently. Therefore, I will not stop until I have."

3. "I am absolutely certain that I can lose this weight. All it takes is time and effort."

Repeat these sentences, or others like them, to yourself during the day, but especially around meal times when you can make the explicit connection between present behavior and future goal. These variations in your theme of faith will stimulate your imagination and, therefore, your desire to win.

*When you get into
a tight place
and everything goes
against you until
it seems you cannot
hold on a minute longer,
never give up then,
for that is just
the place and time
that the tide will turn.
Success is endurance
for one moment more.*

—Harriet Beecher Stowe

Seven Ways to Build Dieting Persistence

What's the difference between the dieter who continually tries to diet and fails, and the kind of dieter who steadfastly sticks to his diet through good times and bad; the dieter who carries on despite demoralizing setbacks and temporary defeats and carries his efforts through thick and thin forever?

Is it physical or moral superiority? Is it finding the "right" diet? Is it unflagging support from family and close friends? Is it luck? Or is it an unremitting will to win?

While you could argue that all of these qualities are important, most people would agree that one singular trait propels more dieters into winners' circles than all others combined. That quality is *persistence*.

Persistence suggests a determined enthusiasm that refuses to be compromised. It indicates a lack of self-pity or self-indulgence. And it implies above all else that unyielding "will to win," a refusal to surrender despite petty annoyances, major obstacles, even demoralizing setbacks.

Call it tenacity, stamina, guts, or determination, this uniquely human trait translates into that enviable quality of hanging on until victory has been achieved. The winners we see and admire in all walks of life have this kind of willpower. And the winners in the dieting game have it, too.

Lack of persistence is the leading cause of all failure,

particularly dieting. It is, without question, the *sine qua non* of willpower. I know you want to be thin, but do you want it *bad enough* to persist in your efforts—regardless of obstacles—to achieve it?

My experience with men and women who have tried to kick their unhealthy habits has proved that lack of persistence is a weakness that is common to the majority of them. They are ready to give up at the first hint of discomfort or pain. They

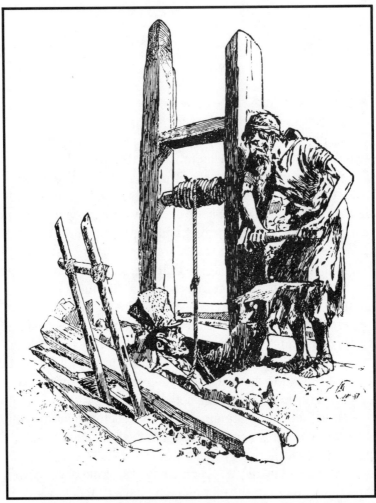

"I always wondered where those fad diets came from."

are easily overcome by delays or setbacks. Only a precious few carry on despite all opposition until they achieve their elusive goal.

Strangely enough, it's just at that point that most dieters could win the weight-loss battle. They only need that little extra willpower to hang on for a short time longer.

This thought was voiced nicely by Greek historian Polybius who said, "Some men give up their designs when they have almost reached the goal; while others, on the contrary, obtain a victory by exerting, at the last moment, more vigorous efforts than before."

Persistent dieters earn their success at just the point where other dieters end in failure. And history is laced with examples where men and women have fallen short of their goal only because they failed to hang on.

How to Spot Weak Persistence

Take a look at your own dieting history. I'm certain that you've been victimized by lack of persistence on many of your previous dieting attempts. It has attacked all dieters at one time or another, often showing up in your dieting life in a variety of disguises. Here are just a few:

1. A willingness, even an eagerness, to succumb to a temporary dieting slip

This is the dieter who uses the occasion of a trifling dieting slip as license for whole-hog bingeing. "What the heck," these dieters say, "I've blown my diet now, so who cares? I might just as well go on eating."

What dieters don't often know is that they set themselves up for most of this wholesale cheating when they fail to surrender to their diet. They carry around the burden of conflicting goals which clash with each other like kids arguing over which TV program to watch. You've already read a great deal about that in Chapter 4 so you know what I mean.

2. The habit of blaming the diet for your inability to stick to a diet or lose weight

As I've said all along in this book, it's not the diet that's at fault when you start cheating again. It's your lack of a well-trained and organized willpower. And there's little sense in blaming the diet since the responsibility is clearly yours.

3. An indifference to meet head-on those situations which we know present great difficulty

Thanksgiving, Easter, Christmas, and all those "bingeing" holidays are troublesome times for dieters, particularly those who haven't made up their minds to meet them head-on and create viable programs for sticking to their diet, despite the obvious temptations.

It's easy to throw up your hands and plead no contest. But dieters who have well-developed willpower know the real world goes on. There will *always* be occasions when "pigging out" seems ritual. So what are you going to do about them?

4. The habit of compromising your dieting goals

If you want to weigh 110 pounds and wear a size three dress, then by all means stick to your diet until you reach your goal. Dieters who lack persistence are willing to settle for something less than what they really want. They've grown weary of diets and long for the time when they can relax and be "themselves" again.

5. Failure to set definite, realistic goals

Nothing leads dieters to failure more often than an ill-designed, ill-advised goal. Although the magazine ads in grocery store tabloids talk about losing ten pounds a week by taking a few pills, it is impossible to lose fat at anything but the going rate: 3,500 calories per pound. So whether you exercise it off or restrain your eating habits, remember there are no free rides when you want to lose weight.

6. Failure to prepare organized plans to achieve dieting goals

Dieters are forever letting other people do their planning. Now it's time to do it yourself. What are you going to do, for example, when you fall victim to a midnight urge for a dish of ice cream? Walk around the block? Watch TV? Take a sleeping pill? What? You've got to have definite plans to head off these tempting times.

7. An unwillingness to *change* eating behavior

Are you ready to change? Or are you still clinging to the old behavior which got you fat in the first place? What is it that got you in trouble? TV grazing from suppertime to the late

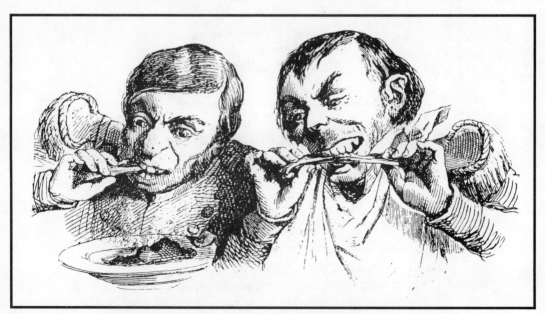

In order to stay thin, you've got to change the way you eat.

news? Too many high-calorie, in-between-meal snacks? Too much of everything at meal times? All of these? Just what is it you'll have to *change?* Are you willing to do so?

HOW TO TEACH YOURSELF TO BE PERSISTENT

Persistence is one aspect of willpower that can be cultivated if you will it to happen. It is based upon eight principles. And here they are:

1. Goal Setting
2. Building Desire
3. Organized Planning
4. Record Keeping
5. Group Memberships
6. Accurate Knowledge
7. The Benefits List
8. Support Activities

Several of these principles have been treated at length in earlier chapters. But for review purposes, let's run through those exercises again.

1. Effective Goal-Setting

Remember? There are five easy rules for effectively setting goals which build willpower:

1. Fix in your mind the exact *goal* you wish to reach.
2. Determine exactly *how* you are going to achieve this goal.
3. Select a *timetable* for the attainment of your goal.

4. Make a *commitment* as to what you'll do to prevent a relapse in your weight-loss program.

5. Reduce your goal statement into *writing* and read it aloud at least three times a day.

2. Building Desire

Desire, as you'll recall, is the motivating force, an emotion, which can be excited to a burning intensity with a series of four exercises. Remember, if you are to be successful at dieting, your desire must be forceful and compelling. You must want to lose weight permanently with enough desire to override the various enemies of dieting such as hunger or depression.

Chapter 6, you'll recall, discussed at length the question of how to build this burning desire. And from your reading you'll remember I prescribed four exercises:

1. Imagination
2. Power Words
3. Reading
4. Keeping Company of Dieting Winners

Continue to do these exercises until you feel you have them down to your satisfaction.

3. Organized Planning

We have also treated in Chapter 7, as part of your plan for effective goal setting, the question of organized planning and why it's necessary to the successful diet. Now all you have to do is keep in mind the lessons you learned through that exercise and put them to use in this one.

Now, however, let's go on to the new exercises.

4. Record Keeping

Accurate record keeping offers you another way to form your own "group conscience" to aid in your persistence. Many dieters and a great many athletes keep diaries, including marathoner Grete Waitz and for exactly this reason.

"The diary," says Waitz, "is important in its function as a

coach, psychiatrist, and conscience. It gives you the opportunity to contemplate your training and to be counseled by it."

When you faithfully keep a dieting (or eating) log, you have important data which can guide your future dieting activities. It gives you knowledge, perspective, and confidence and is a source of dieting motivation.

"A diary is a great inspiration for me," said Waitz. "While preparing for the 1984 Olympic marathon, I frequently looked back to my training the year before for the World Championships, one of my best races. I duplicated the preparation that had given me success, and got added psych by making parallel progress.

"The diary can also simply help get you out the door when you're not motivated," said Waitz, who admits that she, too, has her days when she would just as soon not train. "After all, it's awfully hard to have to write, 'Didn't train today-didn't feel like it.'"

Log Everything in Your Diary

It's very important in this exercise to keep track of *everything*, both good and bad. Obviously, when you're doing well, it's easy to keep records. But when you blow it, you're depressed. And the last thing you want to do is commit that *faux pas* to your permanent record.

But that's exactly what you should do.

Never quit when you're behind! If you have a particularly bad day, record that information just as you do your successful days. This information will serve to bolster your persistence now and at later times because you met the challenge and eventually overcame it.

5. Group Membership

In his book *Think and Grow Rich*, Napoleon Hill speaks often and glowingly of the importance of belonging to a Master Mind Group. "A master mind," says Hill, "is the coordination of knowledge and effort, in a spirit of harmony, between two or more people, for the attainment of a definite purpose."

When two minds get together, a synergy is formed whereby the result is not the sum of two minds, but perhaps three or even more. You not only get ideas from the other person, but you also formulate ideas of your own which you could not have gotten in any other way except through the presence of the other person.

There is a great deal to be said for group membership, particularly when it comes to dieting.

a. Group membership builds confidence. Seeing others succeed plants the seed within you that you can succeed, too.

b. Group membership builds a group conscience. When you share your dieting progress with others, you become motivated by their success. Even their failures, however, can provide important learning experiences by all group members. The group conscience keeps you hustling every week. If *they* can do it, *you* can do it.

c. Group loyalties offer you the opportunity for added rewards when you reach your intermediate goals. Praise is the best diet of all.

d. Group members have knowledge you can get in no other way.

6. Accurate Knowledge: The Dieter's Bill of Rights

Another type of accurate knowledge we need is of the dieting scenario. That's when we familiarize ourselves with what really happens to all successful dieters along their path to freedom from dieting. It's not exactly a bed of roses, but neither is it a briar patch with unfamiliar nettles.

1. Losing weight is a "process" not an act. We need to know that we are going to have dieting slips. That occasional slips are part of the normal *process* of losing weight. It is normal to crave food. More normal still to crave high-calorie food.

2. Losing weight takes time. Two pounds a week is plenty to lose. And when you start talking about three to five pounds,

as the pill peddlers do, you're whistling Dixie. It's possible only the first day or so of your diet until your body gets wise and stops dumping excess water. You just can't sustain a diet with huge daily weight losses. That kind of thinking is for comic books and supermarket tabloids (comics for grownups).

3. Scales are nothing more than approximations. Scales vary. Water weight varies. Internal conditions vary. So don't be tough on yourself. If you gain a pound when you should have lost a pound, remember it's only temporary. The scales of justice will catch up to reality if only you give them time.

4. Dieting has never been easy. To be a winner, you must pay your dues. But whatever hardships you may endure will be temporary. And they'll only add sweetness to your eventual victory.

5. Control is possible. You can weigh whatever you want to weigh. If you want to weigh 145 pounds, you can do it. If you want to weigh 110 pounds, you can weigh that, too.

7. The Benefits List

As a part of Chapter 6 on building willpower intensity, I asked you to put together a list of the benefits which accrue to you as the result of becoming permanently thin.

You may have included some or all of the following:
1. Prettier, or more handsome
2. Younger looking
3. Healthier
4. Longer life
5. Get to wear nicer clothes
6. Clothes look better, wear longer
7. More mobile. You actually can "fit" into a chair
8. Greater stamina. Able to go further, longer
9. Able to participate in sports
10. Able to wear certain fashions
11. Sex is better
12. Sex exists

Now, *every time* you're faced with the urge to quit your diet, I want you to reread your benefits list. Whether you quit or

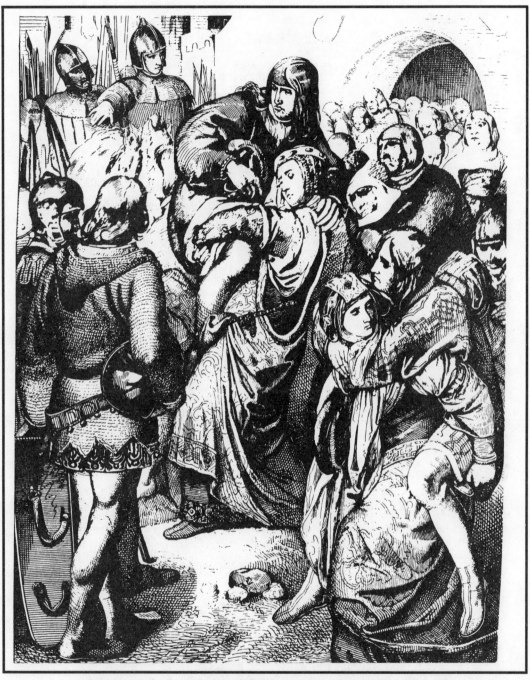

Dieting clubs have learned that one sure way to lose weight is for members to share their burdens.

not. Whether you snitch that cookie or candy or not, *read that list.*

What happens is that soon you'll *automatically* begin seeing that list before your eyes every time you start to cheat. Many times you'll take an alternative action, such as keeping your mouth shut.

8. Supportive Exercise

This book has heretofore mentioned little about the role that exercise plays in permanently losing weight. Since I believe that permanent weight loss is possible only through dieting *and* exercise, I will now give exercising its sweaty due.

> *Your dieting program is doomed to failure unless it incorporates an exercise program.*

As forthright as that statement is, I believe its truth for reasons which are quite different from the usual dieting camp. The "experts" believe the obvious: Exercise burns calories; fewer calories mean fewer excess pounds. I need to quote no medical expert to support this notion. We all know it's true.

A NEW THEORY

But I subscribe to an exercise theory and that's a bit different. I pass it along to you for what it's worth because it exemplifies my sincere belief that anyone can successfully diet if only he puts his willpower to it.

Birds of a Feather . . .

In writing an earlier book, I uncovered an interesting relationship:

> **People who use drugs, use drugs.**

That is, if a person drinks coffee (caffeine), he or she is also more likely to smoke cigarettes (nicotine). And if the person uses caffeine and nicotine, he's much more likely to use alcohol and other drugs as well.

It's an interesting notion that is supported by a wealth of statistical evidence but few, if any, epistomological studies of cause and effect that I'm aware of. Yet, it's accurate enough so that many insurance companies use the relationship to discriminate against certain "drug" users.

Some insurance companies, for example, offer drivers who don't smoke cheaper premiums. They know that smoking in and of itself has little to do with driver safety, save for the occasional hot ash the smoking motorist flicks in his lap.

But smoking has a high statistical correlation with alcohol consumption and, as we all know, drinking and driving means more accidents, injuries, and fatalities. Thus, drivers who don't smoke are a better insurance risk than those who do. And you thought the insurance companies were just being kind to you because you kicked that unhealthy habit.

The theories abound, I suspect, as to why this is true but the "why" doesn't concern us here. What is important for you to consider is that the theory has a practical and effective corollary:

> **People who take care of their bodies will be more inclined to take care of their bodies.**

People who exercise are more likely to be people who don't smoke; people who exercise and don't smoke are much more likely to have normal weights. People who exercise, don't smoke, and have normal weights are more likely to eat balanced, nutritional meals.

Again, I'm not exactly sure why this is true. I just know that it is. By way of an illuminating example, I invite your visual attention to join me at a recent New York City Marathon. It's a cool, cloudy mid-morning in November and the sun futilely tries to cast shadows through the complex spires of the Verrazano-Narrows Bridge.

More than 20,000 eager souls have crushed into an elbow-to-elbow pack almost two city blocks wide and perhaps a half-mile long. Staten Island has become a scientific proving ground for those who want to learn something about fat.

A few runners look absolutely cadaverous. Their bones stick out like jutting knife blades. Their legs look like they'd be better suited to a flock of stilt-legged heron.

But most of the runners throughout this ocean of lean figures are the quintessential definition of being "in shape." They're trim. Solid. Toned. They look every bit as if they could shoulder the ravaging athletic burdens which soon will be thrust upon them.

For in a moment, the thunderous roar from a cannon borrowed from a grassy knoll at nearby Ft. Wadsworth military base will send these agile bodies through a tortuous, 26.2-mile race through the five boroughs of New York to a heaven-sent finish line in Central Park.

As your eyes sweep the panorama of these thousands of men and women, you are suddenly struck by the paradox this sprawling mass of humans represent: More than twenty thousand men and women and not a single cigarette in sight, and overweight runners are as rare as overcoats on Waikiki Beach.

Unbelievable!

I can think of nowhere in the U.S. that this can happen, except at this race in this city. You have to see it to appreciate it: a river of some 20,000 lean and trim bodies coursing through an ocean of two million spectators, at least half of whom have paunches that grow where they should be wearing sweat suits. The visual dichotomy must be seen to be appreciated.

But how does this happen? Well, you could argue that the hundreds of miles a marathoner must run in preparation for such a grueling race makes him or her thin. But you could argue with equal validity that runners are drawn to this kind of athletic competition because they are thin and in excellent physical condition.

Following the same chicken and egg line of thinking, are these runners nonsmokers because they run, or do they run because they are nonsmokers?

Or on another plane, are successful dieters thin because they exercise? Or, do they exercise because they're thin? Or is

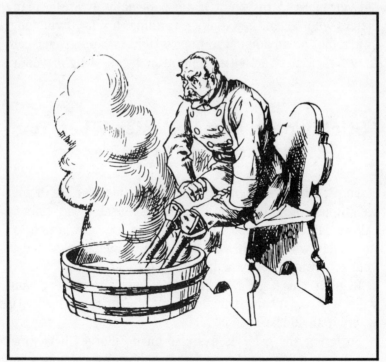

Finisher: 1987 New York Marathon.

147

it, in all of these examples, a little bit of both? One activity begats a spirited participation in the other. And what follows is a sort of self-perpetuating mutual admiration society.

I have no desire to torture this circular reasoning any further because the answer to the enigma is not immediately forthcoming. And yet I do have a theory.

Men and women who begin to take care of their bodies do so in ever-widening spheres. They start small and, buttressed by their success and blossoming willpower, they become (1) interested in, and (2) more capable of, other forms of self-improvement.

I have, for example, personally witnessed many recovering alcoholics who, having achieved a comfortable measure of sobriety, begin a successful program to lose weight, tone up their bodies, quit smoking, and make other salutary improvements to their minds and bodies.

Even more to the point, I am personally aware of many dieters who, when they took up running, hiking, swimming, or aerobics as an adjunct to their weight-loss programs, continued their new activities long after losing weight was an issue.

Sticking to a Diet Is Easier When You Stick to Your Exercises

That's why I recommend that you include exercise in your weight-loss program. Yes, it's an indispensable way to burn calories. But more importantly, exercise has proven to be an invaluable way to help you *stick to your dieting plan* and to your program of permanent weight loss.

Regular exercise is an honest, easy way to keep your willpower to get thin at the forefront of your mental activity, where it should be.

So forget the calories exercise burns. Forget how great you'll look when you tone up that flabby body of yours and coat it with a tan so handsome you'll look like you just made a movie with George Hamilton or Elizabeth Taylor. Just remember this: If you want to stick to your diet, stick to your exercise plan. If you want to stick to your exercise plan, stick to your diet. The two work inextricably well together. When you stick to the one, either one, you'll feel more motivated to stick to the other.

Four Ways to Stick to an Exercise Program

The first thing I'd recommend is that you get yourself a copy of *Rating the Exercises* by Charles T. Kuntzleman and the editors of *Consumer Guide*. Here's a book that compares and evaluates various recreational activities to meet your age, life style, health, and physical condition. It's an invaluable guide to rating what's right for your dieting and exercising needs.

But for here and now, remember that every principle of willpower that I have developed in this book can be applied with equal effect to any exercise program you may undertake.

Since in all likelihood, you have started an exercise plan and failed to stick with it, you may evaluate your reasons for quitting in much the same way as you evaluated your reasons for quitting your diet. Spot the weaknesses in your willpower, and then get to work at strengthening them.

In the meantime, here are some exercising tips:

Choose an interesting activity, one you think you're going to enjoy. If you don't enjoy what you're doing (and give yourself several weeks of honest effort to find out) you won't be able to stick with it. Just keep looking until you find the one that's right for you.

Find the time to regularly practice and develop your activity. For example, many runners and joggers like to hit the trail first thing in the morning because that's the only time they are *sure* they can do their exercises regularly. And as I said earlier, if you're genuinely interested in continuing your exercises, your fitness program comes first. Everything will be assembled around it until you've established that new behavior as habit.

Learn about your sport. If you want to be a runner, buy and read books and magazines about the subject. If tennis is your game, learn all you can. Take lessons. Read books. Join a tennis club. When you get proficient in your sport, you'll like it more, enjoy it more, and stick with it longer. And remember, it takes time to become proficient. So don't write off any activity before you've really given yourself a chance to develop an interest in it.

Set goals and chart your progress. Obviously, one way to know you're getting better, faster, or more accurate, is to keep records. Records are useful yardsticks to measure how far you've come, particularly if you have thoughts about abandoning it later.

Summary

Practice these principles and you'll foster the skill of persistence. Each day you do these and other exercises, you'll find your ability to stick to your diet growing stronger and stronger. Dieting victory will also soon be yours.

*A slave is one who
waits for someone else
to come and
set him free.*

—Ezra Pound

10

Putting It All Together

Now you have all the pieces. Put them together and you've got a plan and program to lift you from the dieting "also-rans" to the winner's circle. By way of a willpower short course, here are some of the highlights of our trip from chapters past.

Willpower is a learned mental ability to control one's behavior through the direction of itself and other psychological forces. There are seven attributes of willpower and each can be strengthened to help you achieve dieting success: decisiveness, strength, desire, concentration, confidence, control, and persistence.

Each reader of this book has in the past skillfully used willpower to achieve significant goals in his or her life. But dieting, apparently, isn't one of them. And that's because when dieters give only partial support to their goals, they use only a partial measure of their willpower. Most frequently they use *strength* of will alone. And to make matters worse, they mistakenly try to use that component to directly control their behavior.

Dieting winners, on the other hand, effectively use all components of their willpower at the right time, in the right proportions, and in the proper way, to produce a favorable result.

Decisiveness, desire, strength, concentration, confidence, and persistence, all have important parts to play in dieting success. The evidence that this is true is about you everywhere. Look at any major project you've successfully completed and notice how you did it. Almost invariably you'll find that you used the full range of your willpower abilities, and most importantly, you evoked these components naturally, effortlessly, to achieve your goal.

This book has shown you how to broaden and unify the various qualities of willpower and how to properly use them. Now it's time to see how this program can work wonders in your dieting life. And to do that, we need a test pilot to walk

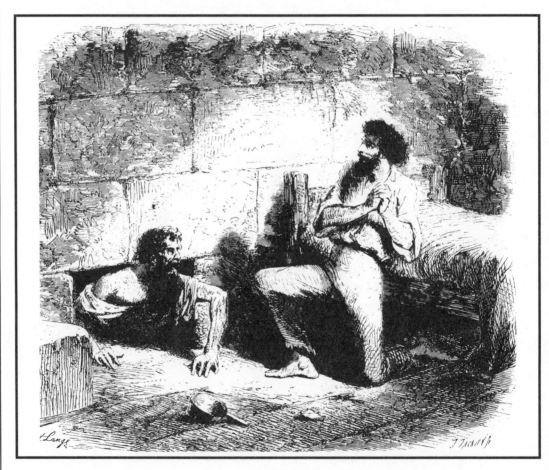

you through the program, somebody who really needs some willpower help.

Ah-ha! Remember Ms. Everydieter of Chapter 1? She had climbed aboard her bathroom scale one fateful morning and found herself an unwilling passenger on a trip to Fat City. She had only one hope: another diet. She's as likely a test pilot as anybody.

But let's assume that Ms. E has been faithfully reading this handy manual and is ready to sprout wings and give it one for the Gipper. It would probably begin something like this:

The Day of Reckoning

One morning after she showers, Ms. E steps to her bathroom scale and discovers, much to her chagrin, that she's gained thirty-seven pounds of ugly, unwanted fat. Naturally, she's disheartened. Crushed. She thought the last time she dieted was going to be the last time. Fat chance. She can now plainly see it wasn't.

But the new Ms. E doesn't make a headlong rush to her bookcase or the corner bookstore to find another dieting panacea. Instead, she produces Wetherall's Ten-Step Willpower Plan for Dieting Success. She reads:

TEN-STEP WILLPOWER PLAN FOR DIETING SUCCESS

1. *Decide to diet*
2. *Set goals properly*
3. *Read appropriate books and magazines*
4. *Keep company with winners*
5. *Develop imagination exercises*
6. *Plan strength exercises*
7. *Build plans for righting wrongs*
8. *Record relevant dieting data*
9. *Remember the benefits list!*
10. *Develop support activities*

Step One

This time Ms. E squarely confronts the issue of whether or not she really wants to diet. Does she really *want* to give up the eating and nonexercising behavior that produced that unwanted fat in the first place?

If she doesn't, she reasons, she might just as well forget it and go have a hot fudge malt for all the success she's going to get. So she takes her time. For the next several days she thinks intently about her state of affairs and the five rules of dieting compliance vs. surrender to test her decision:

1. Is being fat my number one problem? That is, am I willing to put this problem ahead of all others?

2. Will my problem disappear? Do I expect some miracle plan or divine handclap to make my fat vanish?

3. Do I believe that there's only one solution to the dieting problem? Can I honestly admit that eating right and getting sufficient exercise is the one, the *only* solution to my problem?

4. Am I willing to be responsible for getting thin? Or am I waiting for some diet doctor on the *Oprah Winfrey Show* or *Hour Magazine* to find my solution?

5. Will I do anything necessary to become thin? Am I just *saying* I'll stick to an exercise program? Will I stick to an exercise program only so long as I stick to a diet? Will I give up refined sugar if I have to? Will I cut out nighttime TV grazing? Will I *change* my eating behavior? Not just until I reach my ideal weight, but for *good*?

Ms. E sincerely believes she's made the decision to surrender to her diet. But she could be conning herself. After all, she has thought many times before that she "really wanted" to get and stay thin, and yet she has failed every time.

This time, however, she can recognize her previous compliant behavior. She has isolated and identified the compliant nature of her previous dieting performances. All those diets and all those times she was just waiting for them to be over so she could start "eating" again. But no more. Now she's in this for keeps. And she'll find a way or make a way to win her weight-loss battle.

Step Two

Now she's on a roll! And to back her decision she starts setting goals and drafting definitive plans for achieving her goals.

"How many pounds do you want to lose?" she asks herself.

"Thirty-seven pounds," she answers. And Ms. E then gets out her paper and pencil. "How long will it take me to lose them?" she asks. "At two pounds a week that'll take about four months" she figures. But she knows speed isn't really a factor here, since the ultimate goal is not *losing weight*, but building new, thin eating and exercising behavior to make that weight loss permanent.

"How am I going to lose this weight?" she then asks. Ms. E has tried lots of diets. Her best success was with her personal variation of one of the popular "bookstore" diets and she resurrects from her desk drawer her notes on that last dieting attempt.

Next, what about exercise? She's always thought running would be kind of fun so she decides to develop a running program. Not a running program whose viability rests with the continuation of her diet. But a running program which has a separate existence and will continue regardless of the fate of this or any other diet.

Then she asks herself Wetherall's Question: If a person *really wanted* to lose thirty-seven pounds, how would she do it? Not what would *I* do, but what would a person who *really wanted* to lose this weight do?

Couched in these terms, Ms. E goes straight to the heart of the problem free from all the ego-involvement and personal hangups she would experience in prescribing for herself.

"Well, the first thing I think a smart dieter would do," she says, "is find out why she's overweight. If she doesn't know that, she'll never lick the overweight problem once and for all."

When viewed in this way, Ms. E considers a number of alternative answers, two of which she identifies as "her" problem. "I think I'm overweight because I'm always eating after dinner while I watch TV and I never get any exercise." And that behavior, she rightly reasons, has got to go.

The specific solution has yet to be developed. And no doubt she'll try several combinations of different foods, calorie intakes, exercise expenditures, before she finds her final answer. But for now, she's charted a starting point. And so she agrees to cut her daily calorie level to 1,200 and increase her daily exercise level by about 300 calories. And two more things: she also agrees to stop snacking from 6:00 P.M. to 10:00 P.M. and cut out sugary foods entirely.

Step Three

To support her desire to continue her exercise and fledgling running program, she heads for the library. She finds an armload of books on both subjects. For starters she checks out *Diet for a Small Planet* by Frances M. Lappe, *Diet and Nutrition* by Rudolph Ballentine, M.D., *Running Free* by Dr. Joan Ullyot, *World Class* by Grete Waitz, and *Running: The Women's Handbook*, by Liz Sloan and Ann Kramer.

In the coming weeks and months, Ms. E will read her trove of books, enhancing her knowledge of diet, nutrition, and exercise. Each night, time permitting, she selects a chapter or two from one of the books and learns the ropes of how to achieve her intended goal, thus building her desire, her persistence, and her strength of willpower.

Step Four

"That's good for starters," says Ms. E, "but what else would the dieter who really wants to succeed do? Well, she'd probably seek the support of friends, maybe even join a diet club." Righto. Ms. E senses her need to rub shoulders with dieters who are on the winning track. They build her desire, her persistence, her confidence that she can and will succeed. So she starts making plans by adding to her "to do" list.

1. **Check** the Yellow Pages for names of weight-loss clubs. Call Weight-Watchers, TOPS, Overeaters Anonymous, others. Get prices and plans, meeting nights, etc.

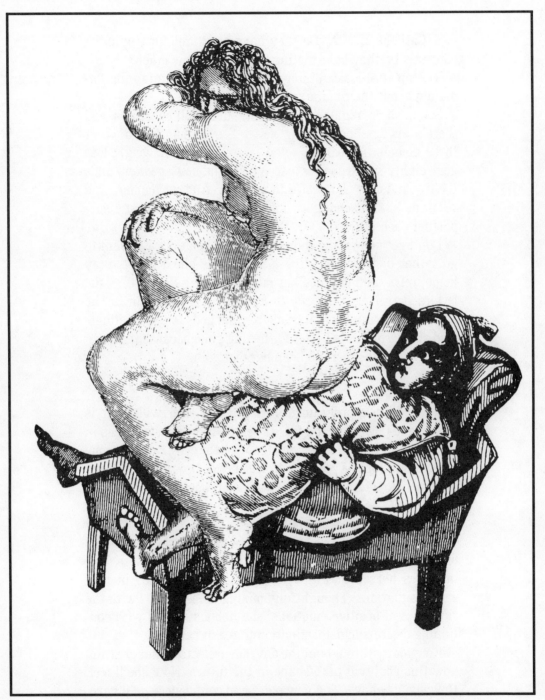

Usually your spouse will let you know when it's time to go on another diet.

2. **Call** the YWCA. Do they have programs for beginning runners? Do they have dieting programs? How much?

3. **Stop** at American Lung Association offices and get information about their running clubs.

Soon, she's regularly attending her club meetings and there's always encouraging news. Steven has lost another three pounds. Barbara is feted for reaching her weight-loss goal: eighty-seven pounds lost. A powerful new speaker builds their confidence and desire to succeed. And newcomers and veterans alike exchange valuable tips and enthusiastic support for each other.

Don't get me wrong, though. Ms. E doesn't always want to go to her diet club meetings. Sometimes she'd like to stay home, relax, and improve her mind watching Vanna turn the letters or reruns of *Eight Is Enough*. But most times she forgoes these intellectual treasures and goes to her meetings. And she *always* feels better for having gone because it consistently works wonders to keep her diet going.

Step Five

Now Ms. E's program is in high gear. Her willpower is strong and powerful. It's fed, as before, by a reservoir deep in memories of her previous gluttonous behavior. But this time she has developed a program to *keep* her desire riding high and forceful. No more does she want her desire and her diet buffeted by the winds of emotional circumstance. She wants to take charge. To *be* in charge.

Each morning before Ms. E leaves her bed, she spends ten or fifteen minutes visualizing her forthcoming success. She imagines herself acting with poise and confidence in new eating situations. Thoughtfully mixing these visuals with the rich hues of positive emotions, she imbues herself with continuing desire and determination to reach her goal.

Frequently throughout the day, she reflects on her goal and how this goal will take shape in the future. How she'll feel. How she'll behave. The new poise and confidence she'll have. And as a result, when she finds herself being enticed by forbidden caloric treats, the images automatically pop into her mind, leading her to a safer shore.

Step Six

But that's not all Ms. E does to head off dieting disaster. To build her strength of willpower, she has regularly been doing things in a way contrary to her previous disposition. She takes the roundabout route when she would have preferred the shortcut. She does later what she wants to do now. She does now what she wants to put off. And each time she performs in a way contrary to her true motive, she develops the skill she needs to say "no" to foods which are contrary to her dieting goal.

But just like every dieter, Ms. E often comes face to face with formidable temptations. But now she's got a tool to extricate herself from what could become a caloric morass. Ms. E opts instead to call on her strength of willpower. "How would someone with strong willpower act in this situation?" she asks. Then she uses her willpower to "act as if" she had strong willpower. Thus, she regains her composure and wins the day.

Step Seven

For the record, Ms. E is not Ms. Mouse, doing a dieting skit straight out of Disneyland. She has a few problems, just like the rest of us. And even though she finds her diet reasonably easy to stick to most of the time, sometimes things go wrong. One day she finds she has not lost the pound she expected, but rather, she has *gained* two pounds. At that moment, the old tapes start playing again, even though she thought they were safely packed away for good. Next thing she knows she marches to the fridge and snatches a carton of ice cream that also should have been packed away someplace for good.

Fortunately, she remembers what Harriet Stowe said. Something like, "When you're in a tough spot, never give up *then*, for that's the time and the place that the tide will turn." And that's just the cue she needed.

"To hell with Harriet," she says, and spoons up a brimming bowlful of Honey Vanilla. "Harriet Stowe never tasted Haagen-Dazs, otherwise she wouldn't have made such a halfwitted remark."

The dish is not even empty yet and Ms. E has begun to get a case of the screaming guilties because of her improvident behavior. The ice cream that she should have removed from its icy vault comes back to haunt her twice over, once when she ate it, again as she tries to rinse the sting of self-reproach-ment from her guilty conscience.

But does she give up? No way. She notes this setback in her logbook and renews her desire to stick to her plan through thick and thin. Ms. E knows that dieting is not a win or lose proposition any more than tennis pros win every game. It's a half-a-dozen steps forward and perhaps one or two back until victory has finally been achieved. And she makes some definite plans on how she'll avoid the ice cream fiasco in the future: *No more sugary treats in this house!* Then she adds that proviso to her goal statement which she continues to read three times daily.

Step Eight

Ms. E realizes that goals are attained a step at a time and these steps can be measured in many ways. To keep track of these various measurements, Ms. E keeps logs. Several of them.

Each day after she showers, for example, she steps onto a scale which is no longer her enemy. And she records her new weight in her dieting diary, her newfound coach and mentor which charts her progress and builds her willpower concentration, confidence, and desire to succeed.

After she runs, she logs how far she went, how fast, and how she felt when her run was done. She compares these data with her goal. Is she on target? Will she have developed her program sufficiently to run the 10-K she promised she'd run in six months? And if she hasn't, what's she going to do about it? Revise her goal? Work harder? Both?

And she keeps tabs on how many willpower exercises she does, too. It's not enough just to do them in the beginning. You've got to keep doing them until you're *successful*.

Step Nine

Like all dieters, Ms. E will be frequently confronted with dieting temptations, large and small. And that's why she always has her Benefits List along—just in case.

She refers to it often throughout the day: before she eats, after she eats, when she's got an idle moment, when she is face to face with ruthless temptations.

At times like these she scans her Benefits List. And she has compiled an impressive list of reasons to tough it out: "More Attractive," she has written. "Sexy," "New Clothes," "New Dates," are among her other personal notations. There's too much at stake for her to flake out now, she agrees with herself. She avoids the temptation. She builds her willpower strength.

Step Ten

Each day as Ms. E marches toward a slimmer figure, she's literally off and running. No big deal here yet. She can only walk and run a half-mile without fear of fallen arches or cardiac arrest. But that's more than she could say when she started. She's on her way toward her first 10-K race which she eagerly awaits although it's still many miles and months away.

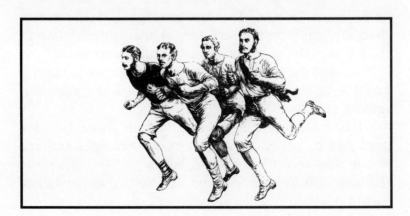

In the meantime, her running program acts as an important catalyst to keep her diet on track. Not only does her body *crave* a better variety of foods, but she is mentally interested in good foods because she truly wants to improve her diet. That is, she knows that when she runs, she is more motivated to eat the kind of foods in the right amounts to improve her running game. And the circle of support is completed. Ms. E knows that as long as she does her willpower exercises, she'll continue to strive for her dieting and exercising goals. And once her new figure is achieved, she'll use her willpower exercises thereafter on only an "as needed" basis.

For All Time

Are you the next Ms. E?

There's no question in my mind that you *can* build an effective will. I have seen dieters and smokers and drinkers make the magic transition from W.I.M.P. (Will In need of Mind Power) to winners, and I know you can do it, too. The only question is whether you truly *want* to do so. If you want to, I know you *can*. But do you want to?

For many dieters, *any* effort is too much effort. I remember distinctly one winter night when I was holding one of my willpower seminars and a woman called me for more information. At conversation's end she allowed as how she would like to come, but couldn't because it was "too cold."

Now I realize it gets cold in Minnesota but the forecast was for an almost "tropical" February overnight low temperature of about twenty degrees and the weather certainly wasn't going to stop the more motivated students from coming.

Obviously, if it was "too inconvenient" to come to class, it would be far too difficult for this woman to do the willpower-building exercises.

If this woman were an isolated example, I wouldn't have mentioned it. But all too often I meet overweight men and women who want to become thin, but only if the goal is easily achieved without sacrifice. And that dieting dream simply doesn't exist.

THE BIG ALIBI

These are the dieters who complain that they "lack" will-power when in fact, they simply don't want to stick to a diet. To cover their corpulent backsides, they invent all sorts of excuses to soothe their consciences and pave the way for continued inability to succeed. See how many of these alibis you have used before:

If only I could find the *right* diet . . .

If my family would only help me . . .

If I didn't have *so much* weight to lose . . .

If I had more willpower . . .

If I could get someone to help me . . .

If I could just get started . . .

If only I weren't so busy . . .

If I had a different job . . .

If I didn't have a family . . .

If I did have a family . . .

If only I wasn't so rushed . . .

If only I could afford to . . .

If someone would invent the magic pill . . .

In the future, write down your excuses here

☐

The Decision Is Yours

The decision is now yours. You can keep on sliding along or you can make the big decision to join the winners, once and for all. You can do it. I know you can.

Don't wait for someone else to set you free. You have the power to grant yourself freedom at any time. The miracle of willing whatever you want is within your grasp right now. All you have to do is summon this awesome power before you and command that it do your bidding.

Heroics are unnecessary. Just do your exercises in small quiet ways and you'll be a winner. Your willpower will learn from these exercises how best to put together a workable team of attributes to accomplish your dieting goal.

This book has the secret you need. The secret of how overweight men and women like yourself shed their excess weight and maintain their leaner, trimmer profiles forever. We have taught you *what* to do, *why* you should do it, and *how* to do it. It is my hope that you will use the techniques I've revealed here and give yourself a lasting and beautiful gift, the gift of the best *you* that you can be. Here's to the winner all of us can be.

Weight Loss through Willpower
DAILY EXERCISE SCHEDULE

WILLPOWER ATTRIBUTE	EXERCISE	REPETITIONS
DECISIVENESS	Reread Chapter 5	____
STRENGTH	1. Doing the Disagreeable	____
	2. Doing It Now	____
	3. Doing It Later	____
	4. Doing Useless Exercises	____
	5. Doing It Your Way	____
	6. Acting as if	____
INTENSITY	1. Imagination	____
	2. Power Words	____
	3. Reading	____
	4. Keeping Company of Winners	____
CONCENTRATION	1. Goal-Setting	____
	2. Change of Attention	____
	3. Focusing on the Dull	____
CONFIDENCE	1. Imagination	____
	2. Repetitions of Goal	____
	3. Words of Power	____
	4. Acting as if	____
PERSISTENCE	1. Goal-Setting	____
	2. Organized Planning	____
	3. Imagination Exercises	____
	4. Record Keeping	____
	5. Group Memberships	____
	6. Accurate Knowledge	____
	7. The Benefits List	____
	8. Supportive Exercise	____

Weight Loss through Willpower
DAILY EXERCISE SCHEDULE

WILLPOWER ATTRIBUTE	EXERCISE	REPETITIONS
DECISIVENESS	Reread Chapter 5	_____
STRENGTH	1. Doing the Disagreeable	_____
	2. Doing It Now	_____
	3. Doing It Later	_____
	4. Doing Useless Exercises	_____
	5. Doing It Your Way	_____
	6. Acting as if	_____
INTENSITY	1. Imagination	_____
	2. Power Words	_____
	3. Reading	_____
	4. Keeping Company of Winners	_____
CONCENTRATION	1. Goal-Setting	_____
	2. Change of Attention	_____
	3. Focusing on the Dull	_____
CONFIDENCE	1. Imagination	_____
	2. Repetitions of Goal	_____
	3. Words of Power	_____
	4. Acting as if	_____
PERSISTENCE	1. Goal-Setting	_____
	2. Organized Planning	_____
	3. Imagination Exercises	_____
	4. Record Keeping	_____
	5. Group Memberships	_____
	6. Accurate Knowledge	_____
	7. The Benefits List	_____
	8. Supportive Exercise	_____

Weight Loss through Willpower
DAILY EXERCISE SCHEDULE

WILLPOWER ATTRIBUTE	EXERCISE	REPETITIONS
DECISIVENESS	Reread Chapter 5	____
STRENGTH	1. Doing the Disagreeable	____
	2. Doing It Now	____
	3. Doing It Later	____
	4. Doing Useless Exercises	____
	5. Doing It Your Way	____
	6. Acting as if	____
INTENSITY	1. Imagination	____
	2. Power Words	____
	3. Reading	____
	4. Keeping Company of Winners	____
CONCENTRATION	1. Goal-Setting	____
	2. Change of Attention	____
	3. Focusing on the Dull	____
CONFIDENCE	1. Imagination	____
	2. Repetitions of Goal	____
	3. Words of Power	____
	4. Acting as if	____
PERSISTENCE	1. Goal-Setting	____
	2. Organized Planning	____
	3. Imagination Exercises	____
	4. Record Keeping	____
	5. Group Memberships	____
	6. Accurate Knowledge	____
	7. The Benefits List	____
	8. Supportive Exercise	____

Weight Loss through Willpower
DAILY EXERCISE SCHEDULE

WILLPOWER ATTRIBUTE	EXERCISE	REPETITIONS
DECISIVENESS	Reread Chapter 5	_____
STRENGTH	1. Doing the Disagreeable	_____
	2. Doing It Now	_____
	3. Doing It Later	_____
	4. Doing Useless Exercises	_____
	5. Doing It Your Way	_____
	6. Acting as if	_____
INTENSITY	1. Imagination	_____
	2. Power Words	_____
	3. Reading	_____
	4. Keeping Company of Winners	_____
CONCENTRATION	1. Goal-Setting	_____
	2. Change of Attention	_____
	3. Focusing on the Dull	_____
CONFIDENCE	1. Imagination	_____
	2. Repetitions of Goal	_____
	3. Words of Power	_____
	4. Acting as if	_____
PERSISTENCE	1. Goal-Setting	_____
	2. Organized Planning	_____
	3. Imagination Exercises	_____
	4. Record Keeping	_____
	5. Group Memberships	_____
	6. Accurate Knowledge	_____
	7. The Benefits List	_____
	8. Supportive Exercise	_____

Weight Loss through Willpower
DAILY EXERCISE SCHEDULE

WILLPOWER ATTRIBUTE	EXERCISE	REPETITIONS
DECISIVENESS	Reread Chapter 5	____
STRENGTH	1. Doing the Disagreeable	____
	2. Doing It Now	____
	3. Doing It Later	____
	4. Doing Useless Exercises	____
	5. Doing It Your Way	____
	6. Acting as if	____
INTENSITY	1. Imagination	____
	2. Power Words	____
	3. Reading	____
	4. Keeping Company of Winners	____
CONCENTRATION	1. Goal-Setting	____
	2. Change of Attention	____
	3. Focusing on the Dull	____
CONFIDENCE	1. Imagination	____
	2. Repetitions of Goal	____
	3. Words of Power	____
	4. Acting as if	____
PERSISTENCE	1. Goal-Setting	____
	2. Organized Planning	____
	3. Imagination Exercises	____
	4. Record Keeping	____
	5. Group Memberships	____
	6. Accurate Knowledge	____
	7. The Benefits List	____
	8. Supportive Exercise	____

Weight Loss through Willpower
DAILY EXERCISE SCHEDULE

WILLPOWER ATTRIBUTE	EXERCISE	REPETITIONS
DECISIVENESS	Reread Chapter 5	____
STRENGTH	1. Doing the Disagreeable	____
	2. Doing It Now	____
	3. Doing It Later	____
	4. Doing Useless Exercises	____
	5. Doing It Your Way	____
	6. Acting as if	____
INTENSITY	1. Imagination	____
	2. Power Words	____
	3. Reading	____
	4. Keeping Company of Winners	____
CONCENTRATION	1. Goal-Setting	____
	2. Change of Attention	____
	3. Focusing on the Dull	____
CONFIDENCE	1. Imagination	____
	2. Repetitions of Goal	____
	3. Words of Power	____
	4. Acting as if	____
PERSISTENCE	1. Goal-Setting	____
	2. Organized Planning	____
	3. Imagination Exercises	____
	4. Record Keeping	____
	5. Group Memberships	____
	6. Accurate Knowledge	____
	7. The Benefits List	____
	8. Supportive Exercise	____

Weight Loss through Willpower
DAILY EXERCISE SCHEDULE

WILLPOWER ATTRIBUTE	EXERCISE	REPETITIONS
DECISIVENESS	Reread Chapter 5	____
STRENGTH	1. Doing the Disagreeable	____
	2. Doing It Now	____
	3. Doing It Later	____
	4. Doing Useless Exercises	____
	5. Doing It Your Way	____
	6. Acting as if	____
INTENSITY	1. Imagination	____
	2. Power Words	____
	3. Reading	____
	4. Keeping Company of Winners	____
CONCENTRATION	1. Goal-Setting	____
	2. Change of Attention	____
	3. Focusing on the Dull	____
CONFIDENCE	1. Imagination	____
	2. Repetitions of Goal	____
	3. Words of Power	____
	4. Acting as if	____
PERSISTENCE	1. Goal-Setting	____
	2. Organized Planning	____
	3. Imagination Exercises	____
	4. Record Keeping	____
	5. Group Memberships	____
	6. Accurate Knowledge	____
	7. The Benefits List	____
	8. Supportive Exercise	____

Weight Loss through Willpower
DAILY EXERCISE SCHEDULE

WILLPOWER ATTRIBUTE	EXERCISE	REPETITIONS
DECISIVENESS	Reread Chapter 5	____
STRENGTH	1. Doing the Disagreeable	____
	2. Doing It Now	____
	3. Doing It Later	____
	4. Doing Useless Exercises	____
	5. Doing It Your Way	____
	6. Acting as if	____
INTENSITY	1. Imagination	____
	2. Power Words	____
	3. Reading	____
	4. Keeping Company of Winners	____
CONCENTRATION	1. Goal-Setting	____
	2. Change of Attention	____
	3. Focusing on the Dull	____
CONFIDENCE	1. Imagination	____
	2. Repetitions of Goal	____
	3. Words of Power	____
	4. Acting as if	____
PERSISTENCE	1. Goal-Setting	____
	2. Organized Planning	____
	3. Imagination Exercises	____
	4. Record Keeping	____
	5. Group Memberships	____
	6. Accurate Knowledge	____
	7. The Benefits List	____
	8. Supportive Exercise	____

Weight Loss through Willpower
DAILY EXERCISE SCHEDULE

WILLPOWER ATTRIBUTE	EXERCISE	REPETITIONS
DECISIVENESS	Reread Chapter 5	____
STRENGTH	1. Doing the Disagreeable	____
	2. Doing It Now	____
	3. Doing It Later	____
	4. Doing Useless Exercises	____
	5. Doing It Your Way	____
	6. Acting as if	____
INTENSITY	1. Imagination	____
	2. Power Words	____
	3. Reading	____
	4. Keeping Company of Winners	____
CONCENTRATION	1. Goal-Setting	____
	2. Change of Attention	____
	3. Focusing on the Dull	____
CONFIDENCE	1. Imagination	____
	2. Repetitions of Goal	____
	3. Words of Power	____
	4. Acting as if	____
PERSISTENCE	1. Goal-Setting	____
	2. Organized Planning	____
	3. Imagination Exercises	____
	4. Record Keeping	____
	5. Group Memberships	____
	6. Accurate Knowledge	____
	7. The Benefits List	____
	8. Supportive Exercise	____

Weight Loss through Willpower
DAILY EXERCISE SCHEDULE

WILLPOWER ATTRIBUTE	EXERCISE	REPETITIONS
DECISIVENESS	Reread Chapter 5	____
STRENGTH	1. Doing the Disagreeable	____
	2. Doing It Now	____
	3. Doing It Later	____
	4. Doing Useless Exercises	____
	5. Doing It Your Way	____
	6. Acting as if	____
INTENSITY	1. Imagination	____
	2. Power Words	____
	3. Reading	____
	4. Keeping Company of Winners	____
CONCENTRATION	1. Goal-Setting	____
	2. Change of Attention	____
	3. Focusing on the Dull	____
CONFIDENCE	1. Imagination	____
	2. Repetitions of Goal	____
	3. Words of Power	____
	4. Acting as if	____
PERSISTENCE	1. Goal-Setting	____
	2. Organized Planning	____
	3. Imagination Exercises	____
	4. Record Keeping	____
	5. Group Memberships	____
	6. Accurate Knowledge	____
	7. The Benefits List	____
	8. Supportive Exercise	____

Weight Loss through Willpower
DAILY EXERCISE SCHEDULE

WILLPOWER ATTRIBUTE	EXERCISE	REPETITIONS
DECISIVENESS	Reread Chapter 5	____
STRENGTH	1. Doing the Disagreeable	____
	2. Doing It Now	____
	3. Doing It Later	____
	4. Doing Useless Exercises	____
	5. Doing It Your Way	____
	6. Acting as if	____
INTENSITY	1. Imagination	____
	2. Power Words	____
	3. Reading	____
	4. Keeping Company of Winners	____
CONCENTRATION	1. Goal-Setting	____
	2. Change of Attention	____
	3. Focusing on the Dull	____
CONFIDENCE	1. Imagination	____
	2. Repetitions of Goal	____
	3. Words of Power	____
	4. Acting as if	____
PERSISTENCE	1. Goal-Setting	____
	2. Organized Planning	____
	3. Imagination Exercises	____
	4. Record Keeping	____
	5. Group Memberships	____
	6. Accurate Knowledge	____
	7. The Benefits List	____
	8. Supportive Exercise	____

Weight Loss through Willpower
DAILY EXERCISE SCHEDULE

WILLPOWER ATTRIBUTE	EXERCISE	REPETITIONS
DECISIVENESS	Reread Chapter 5	____
STRENGTH	1. Doing the Disagreeable	____
	2. Doing It Now	____
	3. Doing It Later	____
	4. Doing Useless Exercises	____
	5. Doing It Your Way	____
	6. Acting as if	____
INTENSITY	1. Imagination	____
	2. Power Words	____
	3. Reading	____
	4. Keeping Company of Winners	____
CONCENTRATION	1. Goal-Setting	____
	2. Change of Attention	____
	3. Focusing on the Dull	____
CONFIDENCE	1. Imagination	____
	2. Repetitions of Goal	____
	3. Words of Power	____
	4. Acting as if	____
PERSISTENCE	1. Goal-Setting	____
	2. Organized Planning	____
	3. Imagination Exercises	____
	4. Record Keeping	____
	5. Group Memberships	____
	6. Accurate Knowledge	____
	7. The Benefits List	____
	8. Supportive Exercise	____

Weight Loss through Willpower
DAILY EXERCISE SCHEDULE

WILLPOWER ATTRIBUTE	EXERCISE	REPETITIONS
DECISIVENESS	Reread Chapter 5	_____
STRENGTH	1. Doing the Disagreeable	_____
	2. Doing It Now	_____
	3. Doing It Later	_____
	4. Doing Useless Exercises	_____
	5. Doing It Your Way	_____
	6. Acting as if	_____
INTENSITY	1. Imagination	_____
	2. Power Words	_____
	3. Reading	_____
	4. Keeping Company of Winners	_____
CONCENTRATION	1. Goal-Setting	_____
	2. Change of Attention	_____
	3. Focusing on the Dull	_____
CONFIDENCE	1. Imagination	_____
	2. Repetitions of Goal	_____
	3. Words of Power	_____
	4. Acting as if	_____
PERSISTENCE	1. Goal-Setting	_____
	2. Organized Planning	_____
	3. Imagination Exercises	_____
	4. Record Keeping	_____
	5. Group Memberships	_____
	6. Accurate Knowledge	_____
	7. The Benefits List	_____
	8. Supportive Exercise	_____

Weight Loss through Willpower
DAILY EXERCISE SCHEDULE

WILLPOWER ATTRIBUTE	EXERCISE	REPETITIONS
DECISIVENESS	Reread Chapter 5	_____
STRENGTH	1. Doing the Disagreeable	_____
	2. Doing It Now	_____
	3. Doing It Later	_____
	4. Doing Useless Exercises	_____
	5. Doing It Your Way	_____
	6. Acting as if	_____
INTENSITY	1. Imagination	_____
	2. Power Words	_____
	3. Reading	_____
	4. Keeping Company of Winners	_____
CONCENTRATION	1. Goal-Setting	_____
	2. Change of Attention	_____
	3. Focusing on the Dull	_____
CONFIDENCE	1. Imagination	_____
	2. Repetitions of Goal	_____
	3. Words of Power	_____
	4. Acting as if	_____
PERSISTENCE	1. Goal-Setting	_____
	2. Organized Planning	_____
	3. Imagination Exercises	_____
	4. Record Keeping	_____
	5. Group Memberships	_____
	6. Accurate Knowledge	_____
	7. The Benefits List	_____
	8. Supportive Exercise	_____